Critical Care Medicine at a Glance

To my wife and children
Richard Leach

Critical Care Medicine at a Glance

RICHARD M. LEACH

MD, FRCP
Consultant Physician and Honorary Senior Lecturer
Department of Critical Care Medicine
Guy's and St Thomas' Hospital Trust and
Guy's, King's and St Thomas' School of Medicine
St Thomas' Hospital
London

With contributions from

JEREMY P.T. WARD

PhD
Professor of Respiratory Cell Physiology
Department of Respiratory Medicine and Allergy
Guy's, King's and St Thomas' School of Medicine
Guy's Campus
London

JAMES T. SYLVESTER

MD
Professor of Pulmonary and Critical Care Medicine
Division of Pulmonary and Critical Care Medicine
Department of Medicine
The Johns Hopkins Medical Institutions
Baltimore MD, USA

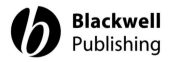

Blackwell
Publishing

First published 2004

3   2008

Library of Congress Cataloging-in-Publication Data

Leach, Richard M., MD.
    Critical care medicine at a glance / Richard M. Leach ; with contributions from James T.
Sylvester, Jeremy P. T. Ward.
        p.   ;   cm.
    Includes index.
    ISBN 978-1-4051-0666-5
    1. Critical care medicine — Handbooks, manuals, etc.
    [DNLM: 1. Critical Care — methods — Handbooks.   WX 39 L434c   2004]
I. Sylvester, James T.   II. Ward, Jeremy P. T.   III. Title.

    RC86.8.L43   2004
    616.02′8 — dc22

                                                                        2004007846

A catalogue record for this title is available from the British Library

Set in 9/11.5 pt Times by SNP Best-set Typesetter Ltd., Hong Kong
Printed and bound in Singapore by Utopia Press Pte Ltd

Commissioning Editor: Vicki Noyes
Managing Editor: Geraldine Jeffers
Editorial Assistant: Nic Ulyatt
Production Editor: Karen Moore
Production Controller: Kate Charman

For further information on Blackwell Publishing, visit our website:
www.blackwellpublishing.com

The publisher's policy is to use permanent paper from mills that operate a sustainable forestry
policy, and which has been manufactured from pulp processed using acid-free and elementary
chlorine-free practices. Furthermore, the publisher ensures that the text paper and cover board
used have met acceptable environmental accreditation standards.

Contents

Preface

Critical care medicine encompasses the clinical skills required for optimal management of severely ill patients in a variety of settings including the intensive care, high dependency, surgical recovery, medical admission, coronary care and emergency departments. It is a discipline that has developed rapidly over the past 30 years and is an essential component of most medical and surgical specialties. Medical students, nursing staff and junior doctors are increasingly required to acquire skills in recognizing and managing critically ill patients by training in such specialist critical care units, and most will be familiar with the sensation of apprehension before starting such training and on arriving in a critical care unit. Unfortunately, most current texts relating to critical care medicine are necessarily extensive. It was our aim in *Critical Care Medicine at a Glance* to provide a brief but rapidly informative text to prepare the 'critical care newcomer' for those aspects of the specialty with which they may not be familiar including fluid management, monitoring, inotropes, sedation, nutrition, airways management, methods of ventilation and end-of-life issues.

As with other volumes in the *At a Glance* series it is based around a two-page spread for each main topic, with figures and text complimenting each other to give an overview of a topic at a glance. Although primarily designed as an introduction to critical care medicine, it may be a useful undergraduate revision aid. However, such a brief text cannot hope to provide a complete guide to clinical practice and postgraduate students are advised that additional reference to more detailed textbooks will aid deeper and wider understanding of the subject. As with many new specialties, certain aspects of critical care medicine are controversial. Where controversy exists we have attempted to highlight differences of opinion, and with the help of colleagues and reviewers to provide a balanced perspective, although on occasions this has been difficult. As with many first editions, errors and omissions may have occurred and these are entirely our responsibility.

Many colleagues have advised and commented on the content of *Critical Care Medicine at a Glance*. We would particularly like to thank our medical associates on the intensive and high dependency care units at St Thomas' and John Hopkin Hospitals and in the Anaesthetics Department at St Thomas' Hospital. Special thanks are due to the senior nurses at St Thomas' Hospital and Clare Leach for advice on the many aspects of nursing care so essential in critical care medicine. Likewise, many students and junior medical staff have acted as 'guinea-pigs', reviewing preliminary chapters and providing invaluable feedback. Finally, we would like to thank all the staff at Blackwell Publishing who have cajoled and assisted us in producing this volume, in particular, Geraldine Jeffers, Fiona Goodgame, Karen Moore and Vicky Pinder.

Richard Leach

Acknowledgements

Some Figures in this book are taken from:

Ward, J.P.T. *et al.* (2002) *The Respiratory System at a Glance.* Blackwell Science, Oxford.

Fig. 48(e) from: Norwitz, E. & Schorge, J. (2001) *Obstetrics and Gynecology at a Glance.* Blackwell Science, Oxford.

Fig. 30 from: O'Callaghan, C. & Brenner, B.M. (2000) *The Kidney at a Glance*, Figs 39 & 40. Blackwell Science, Oxford.

Units, symbols and abbreviations

Units

The medical profession and scientific community generally use SI (Système International) units.

Pressure conversion. SI unit of pressure: 1 pascal (Pa) = 1 N/m². As this is small, in medicine the kPa (= 10^3 Pa) is more commonly used. Note that millimetres of mercury (mmHg) are still the commonest unit for expressing arterial and venous blood pressures, and low pressures—e.g. central venous pressure and intrapleural pressure—are sometimes expressed as centimetres of H_2O (cmH_2O). Blood gas partial pressures are reported by some laboratories in kPa and by some in mmHg, so you need to be familiar with both systems.

$1\,kPa = 7.5\,mmHg = 10.2\,cmH_2O$
$1\,mmHg = 1\,torr = 0.133\,kPa = 1.36\,cmH_2O$
$1\,cmH_2O = 0.098\,kPa = 0.74\,mmHg$
1 standard atmosphere ($\approx$ 1 bar) = 101.3 kPa = 760 mmHg = 1033 cmH_2O

Contents are still commonly expressed per 100 mL (dL^{-1}), and these need to be multiplied by 10 to give the more standard SI unit per litre. Contents are also increasingly being expressed as mmol/L.

For haemoglobin: 1 g/dL = 10 g/L = 0.062 mmol/L
For ideal gases (including oxygen and nitrogen): 1 mmol = 22.4 mL standard temperature and pressure dry (STPD; see Chapter 4)
For non-ideal gases, such as nitrous oxide and carbon dioxide: 1 mmol = 22.25 mL STPD

Symbols

Symbols used in respiratory and cardiovascular physiology are shown in Table 1.

Typical inspired, alveolar and blood gas values in healthy young adults are shown in Table 2. Ranges are given for arterial blood gas values. Mean arterial Po_2 falls with age, and by 60 years is about 11 kPa/82 mmHg. Typical values for lung volumes and other lung function tests are given in Table 3 and *The Respiratory System at a Glance*. Ranges for many values are affected by age, sex and height, as well as by the method of measurement, and hence it is necessary to refer to appropriate nomograms.

Table 1 Standard respiratory symbols

Primary symbols
F = fractional concentration of gas
C = content of a gas in blood
V = volume of a gas
P = pressure or partial pressure
S = saturation of haemoglobin with oxygen
Q = volume of blood

A dot over a letter means a time derivative,
  e.g. $\dot{V}$ = ventilation (L/min)
  $\dot{Q}$ = blood flow (L/min)

Secondary symbols
Gas
I = inspired gas
E = expired gas
A = alveolar gas
D = dead space gas
T = tidal
B = barometric
ET = end-tidal

Blood
a = arterial
v = venous
c = capillary

A dash means mixed or mean, e.g. $\bar{v}$ = mixed venous
A $'$ after a symbol means end, e.g. c$'$ = end-capillary

Tertiary symbols
O_2 = oxygen
CO_2 = carbon dioxide
CO = carbon monoxide

Examples
$\dot{V}o_2$ = oxygen consumption
P_Aco_2 = alveolar partial pressure of carbon dioxide

Table 2 Inspired, alveolar and blood gas values

Inspired Po_2 (dry, sea level)	21 kPa	159 mmHg
Alveolar Po_2	13.3 kPa	100 mmHg
Arterial Po_2	12.5 (11.2–13.9) kPa	94 (84–104) mmHg
A–a Po_2 gradient	<2 kPa	<15 mmHg (greater in elderly)
Oxygen saturation	>97%	
Oxygen content	20 mL/dL	
Inspired Pco_2	0.03 kPa	0.2 mmHg
Alveolar Pco_2	5.3 (4.7–6.1) kPa	40 (35–45) mmHg
Arterial Pco_2	5.3 (4.7–6.1) kPa	40 (35–45) mmHg
Arterial CO_2 content	48 mL/dL	
Arterial [H$^+$] / pH	36–44 nmol/L/ 7.44–7.36	
Resting mixed venous Po_2	5.3 kPa	40 mmHg
Resting mixed venous O_2 content	15 mL/dL	
Resting oxygen saturation	75%	
Resting mixed venous Pco_2	6.1 kPa	46 mmHg
Resting mixed venous CO_2 content	52 mL/dL	
Arterial [HCO_3^-]	24 (21–27) mM	

Table 3 Typical lung volumes for an adult male

Tidal volume (V_T) (at rest)	500 mL
Vital capacity (VC)	5500 mL
Inspiratory reserve volume (IRV)	3300 mL
Expiratory reserve volume (ERV)	1700 mL
Total lung capacity (TLC)	7300 mL
Functional residual capacity (FRC)	3500 mL
Residual volume (RV)	1800 mL

Abbreviations

±	with or without
~	about
A–a gradient	$P_{(A-a)}O_2$ gradient, the difference between alveolar and arterial PO_2
AA	amino acids
ABC	airways, breathing, circulation
ABG	arterial blood gas
ABI	acute bowel ischaemia
AC	activated charcoal
ACE	angiotensin-converting enzyme
ACH	acetylcholine
AChR	acetylcholine receptor
ACT	activated clotting time
ACTH	adrenocorticotrophic hormone
ADH	antidiuretic hormone
AF	atrial flutter; atrial fibrillation
AFE	amniotic fluid embolism
AG	anion gap
AIDS	acquired immunodeficiency syndrome
ALF	acute liver failure
ALI	acute lung injury
ALS	advanced life support
ANA	antinuclear antibodies
ANCA	antineutrophil cytoplasmic antibodies
AP	action potential
AP	anteroposterior
APACHE	acute physiology and chronic health evaluation
APH	antepartum haemorrhage
APPT	activated partial thromboplastin time
ARDS	acute respiratory distress syndrome
ARF	acute renal failure
ASD	atrial septal defect
ATLS	advanced trauma life support
ATN	acute tubular necrosis
ATP	adenosine triphosphate
ATS	American Thoracic Society
AVM	arteriovenous malformation
AVN	atrioventricular node
BE	base excess
BIPAP	bilevel positive pressure ventilation
BIPAP-APRV	BIPAP airways pressure release ventilation
BLS	basic life support
BMR	basal metabolic rate
BP	blood pressure
BPF	bronchopleural fistula
BS	blood sugar
BSA	body surface area
BSD	brainstem death
BSFT	brainstem function test
BTS	British Thoracic Society
CA	coronary artery
cAMP	cyclic adenosine monophosphate
C_aO_2	oxygen content in arterial blood
CAP	community-acquired pneumonia
CBF	cerebral blood flow
CBV	cerebral blood volume
CCB	calcium channel blocker
CCF	congestive cardiac failure
CCM	critical care medicine
CE	cardiac enzymes
CHF	chronic heart failure
CIDP	chronic inflammatory demyelinating polyneuropathy
CK-MB	creatine kinase-MB
CLD	chronic liver disease
CMV	controlled mechanical ventilation
CMV	cytomegalovirus
CN	cyanide
CNS	central nervous system
CO	cardiac output
CO	carbon monoxide
CO_2	carbon dioxide
CO-Hb	carboxyhaemoglobin
COPD	chronic obstructive pulmonary disease
COX	cyclo-oxygenase
CPA	cardiopulmonary arrest
CPAP	continuous positive airways pressure
CPB	cardiopulmonary bypass
CPD-A	citrate, phosphate, dextrose-adenine
CPP	cerebral perfusion pressure
CPR	cardiopulmonary resuscitation
CRF	chronic renal failure
CRP	C-reactive protein
CS	caesarian section
CSF	cerebrospinal fluid
CT	computed tomography
CTT	cardiac troponin T
CVA	cerebrovascular accident
CVC	central venous catheter
C_vO_2	oxygen content in venous blood
CVP	central venous pressure
CVS	cardiovascular system
CXR	chest radiograph
D5%	5% dextrose
DBP	diastolic blood pressure
DC	direct current
DD	diastolic dysfunction
DDAVP	desmopressin acetate or arginine vasopressin
DIC	disseminated intravascular coagulation
DKA	diabetic ketoacidosis
DM	diabetes mellitus
DO_2	global oxygen delivery
DPG	2,3 diphosphoglycerate
DVT	deep venous thrombosis
ECF	extracellular fluid
ECG	electrocardiogram
ECM	external cardiac massage
ECMO	extracorporeal membrane oxygenation
EEG	electroencephalogram
EMD	electromechanical dissociation
EN	enteral nutrition
ER	emergency room
ERCP	endoscopic retrograde choledochopancreatography
ERF	established renal failure
ESR	erythrocyte sedimentation rate
ETI	endotracheal intubation

ETT	endotracheal tube
f	frequency
FDP	fibrinogen degradation product
FEV_1	forced expiratory volume in 1 second
FFP	fresh frozen plasma
F_iO_2	fraction of inspired oxygen
FRC	functional residual capacity
FVC	forced vital capacity
FWB	fresh whole blood
GBS	Guillain–Barré syndrome
GCS	Glasgow Coma Score
GDP	gross domestic product
GFR	glomerular filtration rate
GH	growth hormone
GI	gastrointestinal
GL	gastric lavage
H_2O	water
HAP	hospital-acquired pneumonia
Hb	haemoglobin
HB	heart block
HDU	high dependency unit
HE	hypertensive emergency
HF	heart failure
HHT	hereditary haemorrhagic telangiectasia
HIT	heparin-induced thrombocytopenia
HIV	human immunodeficiency virus
HLA	human leucocyte antigen
HONK	hyperosmolar non-ketotic coma
HpE	hepatic encephalopathy
HR	heart rate
HRS	hepatorenal syndrome
HT	hypertension
HTLV1	human lymphocytic virus 1
HUS	haemolytic–uraemic syndrome
IBD	inflammatory bowel disease
ICF	intracellular fluid
ICH	intracerebral haemorrhage
ICP	intracranial pressure
ICU	intensive care unit
IHA	in-hospital arrest
IHD	ischaemic heart disease
IJV	internal jugular vein
IMA	inferior mesenteric artery
IP	intrathoracic pressure
IPPV	intermittent positive pressure ventilation
ISF	interstitial fluid
ITP	idiopathic thrombocytopenic purpura
LA	left atrial; left atrium
LAP	left atrial pressure
LBBB	left bundle branch block
LC	lung compliance
LDH	lactate dehydrogenase
LMWH	low molecular weight heparin
LRT	lower respiratory tract
LTOD	life-threatening organ damage
LUS	lower uterine segment
LV	left ventricular; left ventricle
LVF	left ventricular failure
MAP	mean arterial pressure
MDMA	methylene dioxymethamphetamine
MG	myasthenia gravis
MH	malignant hyperthermia
MI	myocardial infarction
MILS	manual in-line cervical stabilization
MIP	maximum inspiratory pressure
MOC	myocardial oxygen consumption
MOF	multiorgan failure
MRI	magnetic resonance imaging
MRSA	methicillin-resistant *Staphylococcus aureus*
MV	mechanical ventilation
MW	molecular weight
NAC	N-acetylcysteine
NC	narrow QRS complex
NDI	nephrogenic diabetes insipidus
NG	nasogastric
NIPPV	nasal intermittent positive pressure ventilation
NIV	non-invasive ventilation
NMJ	neuromuscular junction
NMS	neuroleptic malignant syndrome
NO	nitric oxide
NPV	negative pressure ventilation
NS	normal saline
NS	nutritional support
NSAID	non-steroidal anti-inflammatory drug
NYHA	New York Heart Association
O_2	oxygen
OCP	oral contraceptive pill
OER	oxygen extraction ratio
OGD	oesophagogastroduodenoscopy
OHA	out-of-hospital arrest
OT	oxygen therapy
$P_{(A-a)}O_2$	alveolar–arterial oxygen tension difference
P_{50}	Po_2 at which 50% of haemoglobin is saturated
PA	pulmonary artery
P_aCO_2	partial pressure of CO_2 in arterial blood
PAI	primary adrenal insufficiency
P_aO_2	partial pressure of oxygen in arterial blood
P_AO_2	partial pressure of oxygen in the alveolus
PAOP	pulmonary artery occlusion pressure
PAWP	pulmonary artery wedge pressure
PCO_2	partial pressure of CO_2
PCP	*Pneumocystis carinii* pneumonia
PCT	percutaneous tracheostomy
PCV	pressure-controlled ventilation
PCWP	pulmonary capillary wedge pressure
PE	pulmonary embolism
PEA	pulseless electrical activity
PEEP	positive end-expiratory pressure
$PEEP_i$	intrinsic or auto-PEEP
PEFR	peak expiratory flow rate
pH	logarithmic hydrogen ion concentration in arterial blood
PHT	pulmonary hypertension
PiCCO	pulsion continuous cardiac output monitor
PIH	pregnancy-induced hypertension
P_iO_2	partial pressure of inspired oxygen
PIP	peak inspiratory pressure
pK_A	log of the dissociation constant K_A

P_{O_2}	partial pressure of oxygen	SOL	space-occupying lesion
POD	paracetamol overdose	SP	secondary pneumothorax
PP	placenta praevia	SRI	serotonin reuptake inhibitor
PPH	postpartum haemorrhage	SS	scoring system(s)
PPI	proton pump inhibitor	ST	surgical tracheostomy
P_{plat}	plateau pressure	SV	spontaneous ventilation
PRC	packed red cells	SV	stroke volume
PrHT	portal hypertension	$S_v O_2$	mixed venous oxygen saturation
PS	pressure support	SVR	systemic vascular resistance
PSP	primary spontaneous pneumothorax	SVT	supraventricular tachycardia
PSV	pressure support ventilation	SVT/AC	supraventricular tachycardia with abnormal conduction
PT	prothrombin time		
PTCA	percutaneous coronary angioplasty	T3	triiodothyronine
PVD	peripheral vascular disease	T4	thyroxine
PVS	persistent vegetative state	TB	tuberculosis
QOL	quality of life	TC	time constant
Qs/Qt	shunt fraction	TCA	tricyclic antidepressant
Q_T	cardiac output	TDB	third-degree burn
RA	right atrial; right atrium	TE	thromboembolic
RAD	right axis deviation	TII	toxic inhalational injury
RAP	right atrial pressure	TIPS	transjugular intrahepatic portal stent
RBBB	right bundle branch block	TISS	therapeutic intervention scoring system
RES	reticuloendothelial system	TLC	total lung capacity
RF	respiratory failure	TNF	tumour necrosis factor
RFCA	radiofrequency catheter ablation	TP	traumatic pneumothorax
RPC	retained products of conception	TPA	tissue plasminogen activator
RR	respiratory rate	TPN	total parenteral nutrition
RRT	renal replacement therapy	TS	trauma score
RSI	rapid sequence induction	TSH	thyroid-stimulating hormone
RUQ	right upper quadrant	TT	thrombolytic therapy
RV	right ventricular; right ventricle	TTP	thrombotic thrombocytopenic purpura
RV	residual volume	UA	unstable angina
RVF	right ventricular failure	UFH	unfractionated heparin
SA	stable angina	USS	ultrasound scan
SAG-M	saline, adenine, glucose-mannitol	VC	vital capacity
SAH	subarachnoid haemorrhage	VCV	volume-controlled ventilation
SAI	secondary adrenal insufficiency	VF	ventricular fibrillation
SAN	sinoatrial node	VMA	vanillyl mandelic acid
$S_a O_2$	saturation of oxygen in arterial blood	V_{O_2}	global oxygen consumption
SAPS	simplified acute physiology score	V/Q	ventilation/perfusion
SBO	small bowel obstruction	VSD	ventricular septal defect
SBP	spontaneous bacterial peritonitis	V_T	respiratory tidal volume or tidal ventilation
SDB	second-degree burn	VT	ventricular tachycardia
SE	subcutaneous emphysema	VTE	venous thromboembolism
SEMI	subendocardial myocardial infarction	VWD	Von Willebrand's disease
SEp	status epilepticus	WC	wide QRS complex
SIMV	synchronized intermittent mandatory ventilation	WCC	white cell count
		WoB	work of breathing
SIRS	systemic inflammatory response syndrome	WOT	withdrawal of treatment
		WPW	Wolff–Parkinson–White
$S_j O_2$	cerebral oxygen saturation		
SK	streptokinase	Na^+	sodium
SLE	systemic lupus erythematosus	K^+	potassium
SMA	superior mesenteric artery	Ca^{2+}	calcium
SMR	standard mortality ratio (observed mortality ÷ predicted mortality)	Mg^{2+}	magnesium
		Cl^-	chloride
SNPA	soft nasopharyngeal airway	HCO_3^-	bicarbonate
S_{O_2}	haemoglobin saturation		

1 Management of the critically ill patient

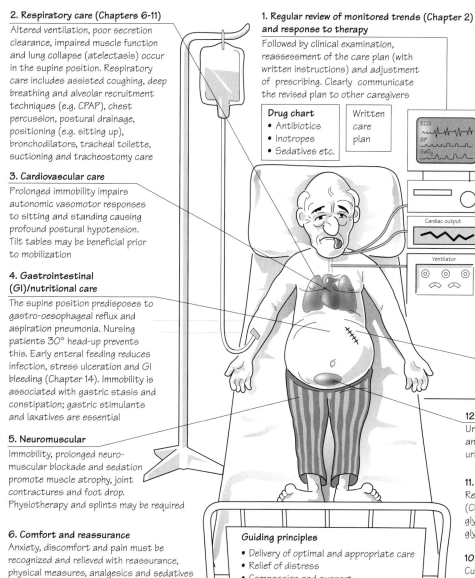

2. Respiratory care (Chapters 6-11)

Altered ventilation, poor secretion clearance, impaired muscle function and lung collapse (atelectasis) occur in the supine position. Respiratory care includes assisted coughing, deep breathing and alveolar recruitment techniques (e.g. CPAP), chest percussion, postural drainage, positioning (e.g. sitting up), bronchodilators, tracheal toilette, suctioning and tracheostomy care

3. Cardiovascular care

Prolonged immobility impairs autonomic vasomotor responses to sitting and standing causing profound postural hypotension. Tilt tables may be beneficial prior to mobilization

4. Gastrointestinal (GI)/nutritional care

The supine position predisposes to gastro-oesophageal reflux and aspiration pneumonia. Nursing patients 30° head-up prevents this. Early enteral feeding reduces infection, stress ulceration and GI bleeding (Chapter 14). Immobility is associated with gastric stasis and constipation; gastric stimulants and laxatives are essential

5. Neuromuscular

Immobility, prolonged neuro-muscular blockade and sedation promote muscle atrophy, joint contractures and foot drop. Physiotherapy and splints may be required

6. Comfort and reassurance

Anxiety, discomfort and pain must be recognized and relieved with reassurance, physical measures, analgesics and sedatives (Chapter 13). In particular, endotracheal or nasogastric tubes, bladder or bowel distension, inflamed line sites, painful joints and urinary catheters often cause discomfort and are often overlooked. Fan use is controversial as dust-borne micro-organisms may be disseminated. Visible clocks help patients maintain circadian rhythms (i.e. day-night patterns)

7. Communication with the patient

Use of amnesic drugs makes repeated explanations and reassurance essential. Assist interaction with appropriate communication aids

8. Venous thrombosis prophylaxis

Trauma, sepsis, surgery and immobility predispose to lower limb thrombosis. Mechanical and pharmacological prophylaxis prevent potentially life-threatening pulmonary embolism (Chapter 27)

1. Regular review of monitored trends (Chapter 2) and response to therapy

Followed by clinical examination, reassessment of the care plan (with written instructions) and adjustment of prescribing. Clearly communicate the revised plan to other caregivers

Drug chart
- Antibiotics
- Inotropes
- Sedatives etc.

Written care plan

ECG
BP
SaO₂

Cardiac output

Ventilator

Guiding principles
- Delivery of optimal and appropriate care
- Relief of distress
- Compassion and support
- Dignity
- Information
- Care and support of relatives and caregivers

15. Visiting hours

Opinions differ with regard to relatives visiting hours. Some units restrict visits (e.g. 2 periods/day), others have almost unrestricted hours

14. Communication with relatives

Family members receive information from many caregivers with different perspectives and knowledge. Critical care teams must aim to be consistent in their assessments and honest about uncertainties. One or two physicians should act as primary contacts. All conversations must be documented. Compassionate care of relatives is always appreciated, avoids anger and is one of the best indicators of a well-functioning unit

13. Dressing and wound care

Replace wound dressings as necessary. Change arterial and central venous catheter dressings every 48-72 h

12. Bladder care

Urinary catheters cause painful urethral ulcers and must be stabilized. Early removal reduces urinary tract infections

11. Fluid, electrolyte and glucose balance

Regularly assess fluid and electrolyte balance (Chapter 5). Insulin resistance and hyper-glycaemia are common but maintaining normo-glycaemia improves outcome (Chapter 32)

10. Skin care, general hygiene and mouthcare

Cutaneous pressure sores are due to local pressure (e.g. bony prominences), friction, malnutrition, oedema, ischaemia and damage related to moist or soiled skin. Turn patients every 2 h and protect susceptible areas. Special beds relieve pressure and assist turning. Mouthcare and general hygiene are essential

9. Infection control

HAND WASHING is vital to prevent transmission of organisms between patients.
DISPOSABLE APRONS are recommended.
STERILE TECHNIQUE (e.g. gloves, masks, gowns, sterile field) is essential for all invasive procedures (e.g. line insertion).
ISOLATION (± negative pressure ventilation) for transmissible infections (e.g. tuberculosis).
THOROUGH CLEANING OF BED SPACES (e.g. routinely and after patient discharge)

In the critically ill patient, assessment of deranged physiology and immediate resuscitation must precede diagnostic considerations. At admission, classification by specialty according to primary organ dysfunction is rarely possible because the history is incomplete, examination inconclusive and diagnosis inadequate. It is this initial diagnostic uncertainty and the need for immediate monitoring and physiological support that defines critical care medicine.

Organization

Critical care medicine (CCM) provides a level of monitoring and treatment to patients with potentially reversible, life-threatening conditions that is not available on general wards. Patients should be managed and moved between areas where staffing and technical support match their severity of illness and clinical needs. Five types of ward area are described: intensive care units (ICUs; level 3); intermediate or high dependency units (HDUs; level 2); admission wards (level 1); general wards; and minimal (or self-care) wards. The principles and practice of CCM encompass ward levels 1–3. Level 3 patients usually require mechanical ventilation or have multiorgan failure. Levels 2 (i.e. medical/surgical HDU, postoperative recovery areas, emergency rooms) and 1 (i.e. acute admission wards, coronary care units) overlap considerably. They provide a high degree of monitoring and support, with level 2 often able to provide non-invasive ventilation or renal replacement therapy. Critical care provision varies from ~2% of hospital beds in the UK to >5–10% in the USA.

Admission and discharge guidelines

These facilitate appropriate use of resources and prevent unnecessary suffering in patients who have no prospect of recovery. Factors determining admission include the primary diagnosis, severity, likely success of treatment, comorbid illness, life expectancy, potential quality of life postdischarge and patient's (relatives') wishes. Age alone should not be a contraindication to admission and every case must be judged on its merit. If there is uncertainty, the patient should be given the benefit of the doubt and active treatment continued until further information is available. Appropriate discharge occurs when patients are physiologically stable and independent of monitoring and support. Out-of-hours and weekend discharges should be avoided, and a detailed handover is essential. In patients with no realistic hope of recovery, and after family consultation, withdrawal of therapy may be considered and organ donation tactfully discussed. Management must always remain positive to ensure death with dignity (Chapter 17).

General supportive care

General supportive care requires a multiskilled team of doctors, nurses, physiotherapists, technicians and other caregivers. The Figure illustrates important aspects of general management in critically ill patients. Prolonged bed rest predisposes to respiratory, cardiovascular (e.g. autonomic failure), neurological (e.g. muscle wasting) and endocrine (e.g. glucose intolerance) problems, fluid and electrolyte imbalance, constipation, infection, venous thrombosis and pressure sores.

Nursing care

The importance of skilled nursing in the management of critically ill patients cannot be overemphasized. Assessment, continuous monitoring, drug administration, comfort (e.g. analgesia, toilette), psychological support, assistance with communication, advocacy, skin care, positioning, feeding, and early detection of complications (e.g. line infection) are vital nursing roles which have a profound effect on outcome. Nurses also provide essential support for relatives, doctors, physiotherapists and other caregivers (e.g. technicians).

Scoring systems

Scoring systems (SS) are used to predict outcome and evaluate care. Two SS have been validated and are widely used in ICUs.

1 APACHE II (acute physiology and chronic health evaluation) aims to measure case-mix and predict outcome in ICU patients *as a group*. It should not be used to predict individual outcome. Scoring is based on the primary disease process, physiological reserve, including age and chronic health history (e.g. chronic liver, cardiovascular, respiratory, renal and immune conditions), and the severity of illness determined from the worst value in the first 24 h of 12 acute physiological variables, including rectal temperature, mean blood pressure (BP), heart rate, respiratory rate (RR), arterial P_aO_2 and pH, serum sodium, potassium and creatinine, haematoocrit, white cell count (WCC) and Glasgow Coma Score (GCS; Chapter 45). Predicted mortality, by diagnosis, has been calculated from large databases, which allows individual units to evaluate their performance against reference ICUs by calculating the standard mortality ratio (SMR = observed mortality ÷ predicted mortality) for each diagnostic group. A high SMR (>1.5) should prompt investigation and management changes for specific conditions.

2 SAPS (simplified acute physiology score) is similar to APACHE II with equivalent accuracy.

Pathology-specific SS are frequently used in CCM.

• **Trauma score (TS)** assesses triage status based on RR, respiratory effort, systolic BP, capillary refill and GCS. A high score indicates the need for transfer to a trauma centre. **Revised TS** uses only GCS, RR and systolic BP with improved prognostic reliability but less suitability for triage.

• **Abbreviated injury scale** assesses multiple injuries and correlates with morbidity and mortality.

• **Other SS** include the paediatric trauma score, neonatal Apgar score and GCS (Chapter 45).

Costs of CCM

Measuring ICU costs is complex. The most widely used system is the **Therapeutic Intervention Scoring System** (TISS), which scores the overall requirements for care by measuring nursing activity and interventions. TISS correlates well with staff, equipment and drug costs and can also be used as an index of nurse dependency. The majority (>50%) of ICU expenditure is on labour costs, in particular constant bedside nursing. Drugs, imaging, laboratory tests and supplies account for ~40% of spending. Consequently, cost saving usually requires personnel reductions, and risks lowering quality of care. Current estimates of daily ('basic') ICU costs vary from £800 to £1600 in the UK. HDU costs are ~50% and general ward care ~20% of ICU costs. In the USA, ~13% of gross domestic product (GDP) is spent on healthcare, with critical care costs ~7% of total expenditure. In comparison, the UK spends ~7–8% of GDP on healthcare with ~1% of total expenditure directed to critical care provision.

2 Monitoring in critical care medicine

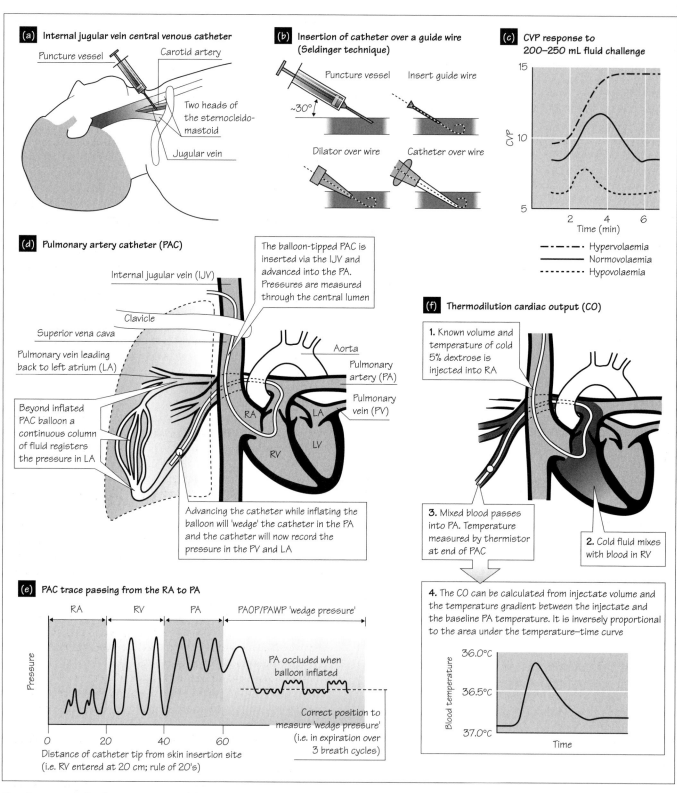

(a) Internal jugular vein central venous catheter

Puncture vessel
Carotid artery
Two heads of the sternocleido-mastoid
Jugular vein

(b) Insertion of catheter over a guide wire (Seldinger technique)

Puncture vessel   Insert guide wire
~30°
Dilator over wire   Catheter over wire

(c) CVP response to 200–250 mL fluid challenge

CVP
15
10
5
Time (min)
2   4   6

– · – · – Hypervolaemia
———— Normovolaemia
········· Hypovolaemia

(d) Pulmonary artery catheter (PAC)

The balloon-tipped PAC is inserted via the IJV and advanced into the PA. Pressures are measured through the central lumen

Internal jugular vein (IJV)
Clavicle
Superior vena cava
Pulmonary vein leading back to left atrium (LA)
Beyond inflated PAC balloon a continuous column of fluid registers the pressure in LA
Aorta
Pulmonary artery (PA)
Pulmonary vein (PV)
RA   LA
RV   LV

Advancing the catheter while inflating the balloon will 'wedge' the catheter in the PA and the catheter will now record the pressure in the PV and LA

(f) Thermodilution cardiac output (CO)

1. Known volume and temperature of cold 5% dextrose is injected into RA

3. Mixed blood passes into PA. Temperature measured by thermistor at end of PAC

2. Cold fluid mixes with blood in RV

4. The CO can be calculated from injectate volume and the temperature gradient between the injectate and the baseline PA temperature. It is inversely proportional to the area under the temperature–time curve

Blood temperature
36.0°C
36.5°C
37.0°C
Time

(e) PAC trace passing from the RA to PA

Pressure
RA   RV   PA   PAOP/PAWP 'wedge pressure'

PA occluded when balloon inflated

Correct position to measure 'wedge pressure' (i.e. in expiration over 3 breath cycles)

0   20   40   60
Distance of catheter tip from skin insertion site (i.e. RV entered at 20 cm; rule of 20's)

Continuous monitoring ensures rapid detection of change in clinical parameters and accurate assessment of progress and response to therapy. The following principles apply.

• **Monitoring is an aid to assessment.** Regular clinical examination is essential. Simple physical signs, such as appearance, peripheral perfusion (e.g. cold, pale skin) and conscious level, are as important as parameters displayed on a monitor. When clinical signs and monitored parameters disagree, *assume that clinical* *assessment is correct*, until potential errors from the monitored variable have been excluded (e.g. incorrect CVP reading due to blocked lines or incorrect calibration). **Trends** are generally more important than single readings.

- **Use non-invasive techniques whenever possible** as invasive methods are associated with potential risks (e.g. line infection) and complications (e.g. pneumothorax). Always ask 'Is an invasive technique necessary?' and replace it with a non-invasive method as soon as possible. **Alarms** are a crucial safety feature (e.g. ventilator disconnection in a paralysed patient). They are set to physiological safe limits and should never be disconnected.

Haemodynamic monitoring

Blood pressure (BP) is often measured intermittently using an automated sphygmomanometer. In critically ill patients continuous intra-arterial monitoring is preferred. It must be appreciated that BP does not reflect cardiac output (CO). Thus, BP can be normal or high, but CO low, when generalized vasoconstriction raises systemic vascular resistance (SVR). Conversely, the vasodilated, 'septic' patient with low SVR may be hypotensive despite a high CO (Chapters 4 and 16).

Central venous pressure (CVP) is measured using internal jugular (Figs a and b) or subclavian vein catheters and reflects the right atrial pressure (RAP). It is a useful means of assessing circulating blood volume and determining the rate at which fluid should be administered. However, during hypovolaemia or haemorrhage (i.e. low CVP expected), increased venous tone can act to maintain CVP and mask volume depletion. Consequently, in this situation, CVP measurement is not as important as **the response to a fluid challenge** (Fig. c). A high CVP indicates excessive intravascular volume, impaired myocardial contractility or increased right ventricular afterload. Management depends on the cause (Chapters 4, 20).

Pulmonary artery wedge/occlusion pressure (PAWP/PAOP) reflects left atrial pressure (LAP). Normally CVP is an adequate guide to filling pressures on both sides of the heart, but in critical illness and ischaemic heart disease (IHD) there may be a 'disparity' between left and right ventricular function. For example, low RAP may occur with high LAP in left ventricular dysfunction. Small rises in RAP can cause large LAP increases which may precipitate pulmonary oedema (Chapter 20). In these situations, PAWP is monitored using a pulmonary artery (PA) catheter (Figs d and e). PAWP is normally 6–12 mmHg, but in left ventricular failure (LVF) may be > 25–35 mmHg. Provided the pulmonary capillary membranes are intact (i.e. not 'leaky'), a PAWP of ~15 mmHg ensures good left ventricular filling and optimal function without risking pulmonary oedema. PA catheters also measure cardiac output, mixed venous saturation and right ventricular (RV) ejection fraction (see below).

Cardiac output (CO) is usually measured by thermodilution (Fig. f; e.g. PA catheter, pulsion continuous cardiac output monitor (PiCCO)). Although this is often regarded as the gold standard for CO measurement, the error is at least 10%. Non- (or less) invasive techniques of CO monitoring utilize dye/lithium dilution, transoesophageal Doppler ultrasonography, echocardiography or impedance methods.

Electrocardiogram (ECG). Rate and rhythm are displayed by standard single-lead ECG monitors but ST segment changes can be monitored in patients with IHD.

Respiratory monitoring

Arterial blood gases monitor P_aO_2, P_aCO_2 and acid–base balance. Measurement aids diagnosis and allows adjustment of ventilation to achieve optimum gas exchange (Chapters 6, 10, 12).

Arterial oxygen saturation (S_aO_2) is determined by spectrophotometric analysis of the proportion of saturated to desaturated haemoglobin. Commonly used finger or earlobe probes are unreliable if peripheral perfusion is poor. Oxygenation is usually adequate if S_aO_2 is >90%.

Mixed venous oxygen saturation (S_vO_2) is measured using fibreoptic PA catheters or PA blood sampling and co-oximetry. It is normally >65–70%. A low S_vO_2 (<55–60%) may indicate inadequate tissue O_2 delivery even when S_aO_2 and P_aO_2 are normal (e.g. cardiac failure, anaemia).

Lung function. Alveolar–arterial PO_2 gradient and P_aO_2/F_iO_2 ratio are measures of gas exchange. Arterial and end-tidal CO_2 (see below) indicate adequacy of alveolar ventilation. Peak expiratory flow rate (PEFR) and spirometric changes in forced expiratory volume in 1 second (FEV_1) and vital capacity (VC) are often monitored in self-ventilating patients with lung disease (Chapters 24, 25). Maximum inspiratory pressure (MIP) in an intubated patient is normally ~100 cmH$_2$O. An MIP < 25 cmH$_2$O indicates that spontaneous ventilation following extubation is unlikely (e.g. due to muscle weakness).

Lung compliance (LC) is the tidal ventilation (V_T; mL) divided by the pressure (cmH$_2$O) required to achieve V_T. It is a measure of lung 'stiffness' or ease of inflation and is reduced in damaged lungs. High airways pressures during mechanical ventilation indicate reduced LC.

Capnography. Inspired air contains virtually no CO_2. At the end of expiration, the end-tidal CO_2 concentration closely mirrors arterial P_aCO_2 and indicates the adequacy of alveolar ventilation provided the distribution of ventilation is uniform.

Organ and tissue oxygenation

Global measures (e.g. S_vO_2, lactate) reflect the adequacy of total tissue perfusion but may be normal despite severe regional perfusion abnormalities. Increased serial lactate concentrations and metabolic acidosis suggest anaerobic metabolism and inadequate tissue oxygenation. However, lactate may increase in the absence of hypoxia (e.g. liver failure, sepsis). An S_vO_2 < 55% indicates global tissue hypoxia.

Organ-specific measures include:

- **urine flow** which is a sensitive measure of renal perfusion (Chapter 30) provided that the kidneys are not damaged (e.g. acute tubular necrosis) or affected by drugs (e.g. diuretics). Hourly urine output is normally ~1 mL/kg
- **core–peripheral temperature,** the gradient between peripheral (e.g. skin temperature over the dorsum of the foot) and core temperature (e.g. rectal, oesophageal), is often used as an index of peripheral perfusion
- **gastric tonometry** which is occasionally used to detect shock-induced splanchnic ischaemia by measuring gastric luminal PCO_2 and subsequently deriving mucosal pH
- **neurological monitoring** which utilizes the Glasgow Coma Score, intracranial pressure measurement and jugular venous bulb saturation (Chapter 45).

3 Oxygen transport

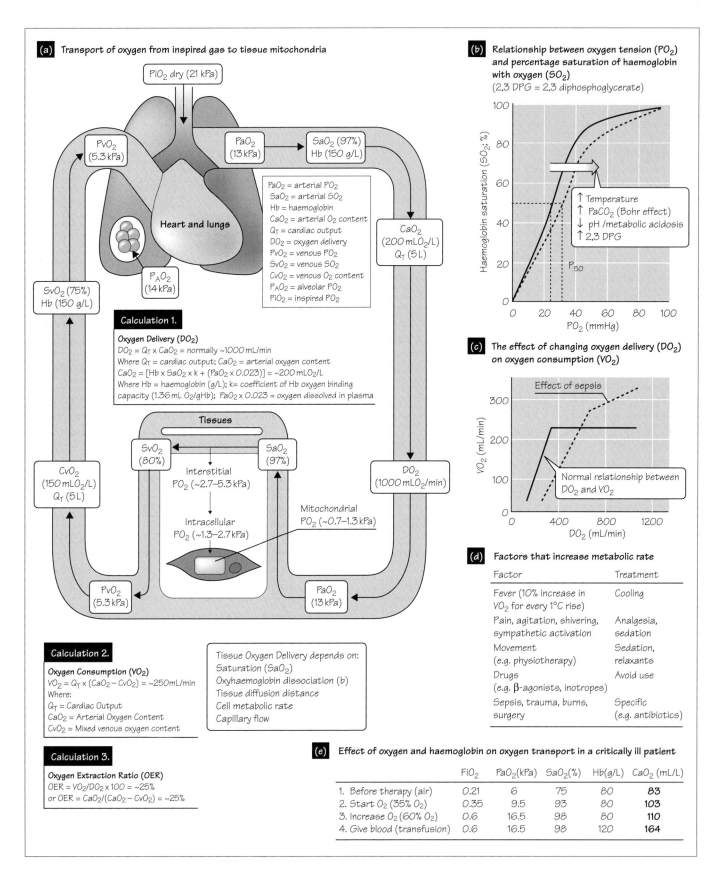

(a) Transport of oxygen from inspired gas to tissue mitochondria

PiO₂ dry (21 kPa)

PvO₂ (5.3 kPa)

PaO₂ (13 kPa)

SaO₂ (97%) Hb (150 g/L)

Heart and lungs

PaO₂ = arterial PO₂
SaO₂ = arterial SO₂
Hb = haemoglobin
CaO₂ = arterial O₂ content
Qₜ = cardiac output
DO₂ = oxygen delivery
PvO₂ = venous PO₂
SvO₂ = venous SO₂
CvO₂ = venous O₂ content
PₐO₂ = alveolar PO₂
PiO₂ = inspired PO₂

CaO₂ (200 mLO₂/L) Qₜ (5 L)

PₐO₂ (14 kPa)

SvO₂ (75%) Hb (150 g/L)

Calculation 1.

Oxygen Delivery (DO₂)
DO₂ = Qₜ × CaO₂ = normally ~1000 mL/min
Where Qₜ = cardiac output; CaO₂ = arterial oxygen content
CaO₂ = [Hb × SaO₂ × k + (PaO₂ × 0.023)] = ~200 mLO₂/L
Where Hb = haemoglobin (g/L); k= coefficient of Hb oxygen binding
capacity (1.36 mL O₂/gHb); PaO₂ × 0.023 = oxygen dissolved in plasma

Tissues

SvO₂ (80%)

SaO₂ (97%)

Interstitial PO₂ (~2.7–5.3 kPa)

Intracellular PO₂ (~1.3–2.7 kPa)

Mitochondrial PO₂ (~0.7–1.3 kPa)

CvO₂ (150 mLO₂/L) Qₜ (5 L)

DO₂ (1000 mLO₂/min)

PvO₂ (5.3 kPa)

PaO₂ (13 kPa)

Calculation 2.

Oxygen Consumption (VO₂)
VO₂ = Qₜ × (CaO₂ – CvO₂) = ~250mL/min
Where:
Qₜ = Cardiac Output
CaO₂ = Arterial Oxygen Content
CvO₂ = Mixed venous oxygen content

Tissue Oxygen Delivery depends on:
Saturation (SaO₂)
Oxyhaemoglobin dissociation (b)
Tissue diffusion distance
Cell metabolic rate
Capillary flow

Calculation 3.

Oxygen Extraction Ratio (OER)
OER = VO₂/DO₂ × 100 = ~25%
or OER = CaO₂/(CaO₂ – CvO₂) = ~25%

(b) Relationship between oxygen tension (PO₂) and percentage saturation of haemoglobin with oxygen (SO₂)
(2,3 DPG = 2,3 diphosphoglycerate)

↑ Temperature
↑ PaCO₂ (Bohr effect)
↓ pH /metabolic acidosis
↑ 2,3 DPG

P₅₀

Haemoglobin saturation (SO₂; %)
PO₂ (mmHg)

(c) The effect of changing oxygen delivery (DO₂) on oxygen consumption (VO₂)

Effect of sepsis

Normal relationship between DO₂ and VO₂

VO₂ (mL/min)
DO₂ (mL/min)

(d) Factors that increase metabolic rate

Factor	Treatment
Fever (10% increase in VO₂ for every 1°C rise)	Cooling
Pain, agitation, shivering, sympathetic activation	Analgesia, sedation
Movement (e.g. physiotherapy)	Sedation, relaxants
Drugs (e.g. β-agonists, inotropes)	Avoid use
Sepsis, trauma, burns, surgery	Specific (e.g. antibiotics)

(e) Effect of oxygen and haemoglobin on oxygen transport in a critically ill patient

	FiO₂	PaO₂(kPa)	SaO₂(%)	Hb(g/L)	CaO₂ (mL/L)
1. Before therapy (air)	0.21	6	75	80	83
2. Start O₂ (35% O₂)	0.35	9.5	93	80	103
3. Increase O₂ (60% O₂)	0.6	16.5	98	80	110
4. Give blood (transfusion)	0.6	16.5	98	120	164

The major function of the heart, lungs and circulation is to provide oxygen and other nutrients to body tissues and remove carbon dioxide and other waste products of metabolism. The determinants of oxygen transport are:

1 *loading of blood with oxygen in the lungs*, measured by the arterial oxygen content (C_aO_2) and determined by alveolar oxygen (P_AO_2), efficiency of lung oxygen exchange, blood haemoglobin (Hb) content and the oxyhaemoglobin dissociation curve;

2 *convective oxygen transport from the lungs to the tissues*, determined (after oxygen loading in the lungs) by the magnitude and regional distribution of cardiac output (Q_T); and

3 *diffusional oxygen transport from capillary blood to tissue mitochondria*, determined by the capillary–mitochondrial PO_2 gradient, capillary surface area and diffusion distance.

Controls at each stage usually ensure that oxygen utilization is not limited by transport.

Oxygen delivery

Figure (a) illustrates the transport of oxygen from inspired air to tissue mitochondria.

- **Global oxygen delivery (DO_2)** is determined from Q_T and C_aO_2 (Fig. a; Calculation 1). Most oxygen carried in blood is attached to Hb. Only a small amount is dissolved in plasma. Arterial oxygen saturation (S_aO_2) and Hb concentration are the major determinants of C_aO_2. Figure (e) illustrates the relative effects of increasing oxygen and Hb on DO_2. Although transfusion rapidly increases DO_2, the optimum Hb level in critical illness is ~100 g/L (10 g/dL) and is a balance between optimizing the C_aO_2 and avoiding microcirculatory problems due to viscosity. Fluid administration and inotropes are used to increase Q_T and DO_2 (Chapter 5). However, a high DO_2 will not prevent death due to severe single-organ ischaemia (e.g. mesenteric arterial embolus). In this situation, only removal of the local obstruction to blood flow is life-saving (e.g. embolectomy).

- **Tissue oxygen delivery** requires appropriate regional and microcirculatory distribution of Q_T, which is determined by a complex interaction of endothelial, receptor, metabolic and pharmacological factors. During stress or critical illness, blood flow is directed to vital organs (e.g. brain) and away from less essential tissue beds (e.g. splanchnic, skin) which are damaged if this effect persists. For example, prolonged splanchnic ischaemia compromises bowel wall integrity, causing translocation of bacteria into the circulation. Therapeutically, receptor properties of certain vasoactive agents can be used to improve individual organ oxygen delivery (e.g. dopexamine increases splanchnic blood flow).

- **Tissue factors** influence cellular oxygen status. Oxygen diffuses from the capillary to the cell and is dependent on capillary blood flow and surface area (i.e. reduced by capillary thrombosis), oxygen gradient and diffusion distance. However, increasing DO_2 cannot compensate for cellular metabolic failure (e.g. mitochondrial dysfunction during sepsis). In addition, some tissues (e.g. brain, kidney) are more susceptible to, and are rapidly damaged by, sustained hypoxia.

The oxyhaemoglobin dissociation curve

Figure (b) illustrates the relationship between the partial pressure of oxygen (PO_2) in the blood and Hb saturation (SO_2). The position of the dissociation curve is affected by temperature, pH, P_aCO_2 and 2,3 diphosphoglycerate (DPG), and is measured by the PO_2 at which 50% of the Hb is saturated (P_{50}). This is normally 3.5 kPa (26 mmHg). Left or right shifts of the curve will alter uptake and release of oxygen by the Hb molecule. If the curve moves to the right, the S_aO_2 will be lower for a given PO_2 (i.e. less oxygen will be taken up in the lungs but more will be released in the tissues). Thus, as capillary PCO_2 increases (i.e. rightward shift of the curve), oxygen is released from Hb, a phenomenon known as the Bohr effect.

Oxygen consumption

- **Global oxygen consumption (VO_2)** is the sum of the oxygen consumed by individual organs and tissues and is ~250 mL/min for a 70-kg adult. It can be calculated from Q_T, S_aO_2 and S_vO_2 (Fig. a; Calculation 2) or from the inspired and mixed expired oxygen and CO_2 concentrations. The oxygen extraction ratio (OER; Fig. a; Calculation 3) determines the amount of oxygen used (VO_2) as a percentage of that delivered (DO_2) and is normally ~25%.

- **Metabolic rate.** Factors that increase metabolic rate are listed in Fig. (d). It should be recognized that drugs used to increase DO_2 (e.g. inotropes) may also increase VO_2. Simple measures including cooling, analgesia, sedation, prevention of shivering and muscle relaxation substantially reduce VO_2 and subsequent DO_2 requirements.

Relationship between oxygen delivery (DO_2) and oxygen consumption (VO_2)

Figure (c) illustrates the effect of changing DO_2 on VO_2 in normal and septic patients. Normally oxygen extraction from capillary blood increases as tissue consumption rises or blood supply decreases. The maximum OER is about 70%. Any further increase in tissue oxygen consumption or fall in oxygen supply will result in hypoxia, anaerobic metabolism and lactic acid production. In this situation, DO_2 must be improved by increasing oxygenated blood flow to the tissue or relieving obstruction (e.g. thrombolysis in myocardial infarction).

In sepsis, cellular dysfunction reduces the ability of tissues to extract oxygen. This alters the relationship between DO_2 and VO_2 (Fig. c). In particular, VO_2 continues to increase even at 'supranormal' levels of DO_2. This observation encouraged the use of aggressive fluid loading and inotropic support to achieve high oxygen deliveries (>600 mL/min/m^2), in the belief that this strategy, sometimes termed **goal-directed therapy**, would relieve hypoxia and prevent tissue damage. However, this has not been demonstrated to be the case. Microcirculatory impairment (i.e. capillary thrombi), failure of regional distribution and metabolic dysfunction are more likely than inadequate DO_2 to cause cellular toxicity in late sepsis.

Venous blood saturation varies according to the metabolic requirements of individual tissues (i.e. hepatic 30–40%, renal ~80%). In the pulmonary artery, the **mixed venous oxygen saturation** ($S_vO_2 > 65$–70%) represents the oxygen not used in the tissues ($DO_2 - VO_2$). It is influenced by both DO_2 and VO_2 and, provided regional blood flow and cellular oxygen utilization are normal, can be used to reflect whether global DO_2 is adequately matching global VO_2 (Chapter 2).

4 Shock

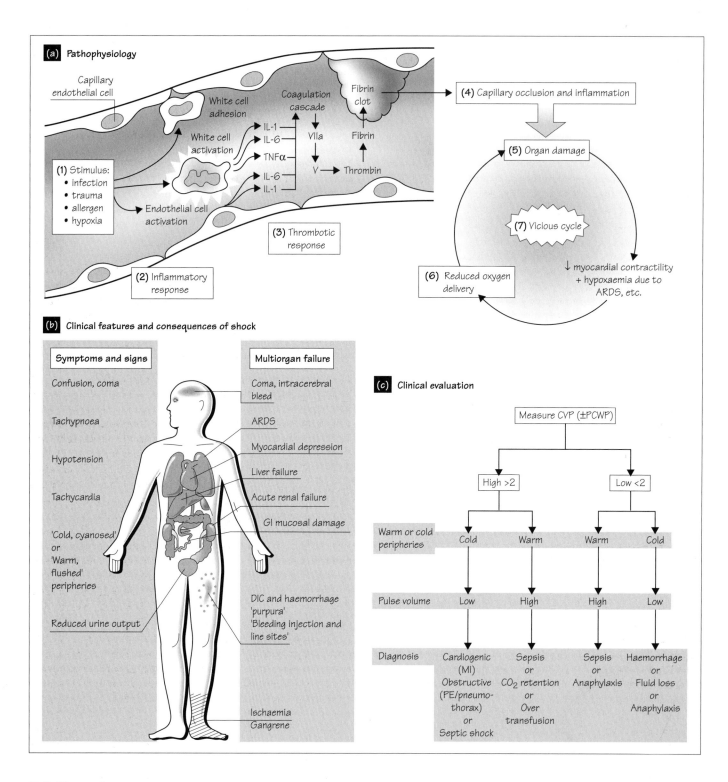

(a) Pathophysiology

Capillary endothelial cell

White cell adhesion

White cell activation

(1) Stimulus:
- infection
- trauma
- allergen
- hypoxia

Endothelial cell activation

Coagulation cascade

IL-1
IL-6
TNFα
IL-6
IL-1

VIIa → Fibrin
V → Thrombin → Fibrin

Fibrin clot

(4) Capillary occlusion and inflammation

(5) Organ damage

(7) Vicious cycle

↓ myocardial contractility + hypoxaemia due to ARDS, etc.

(6) Reduced oxygen delivery

(3) Thrombotic response

(2) Inflammatory response

(b) Clinical features and consequences of shock

Symptoms and signs	Multiorgan failure
Confusion, coma	Coma, intracerebral bleed
Tachypnoea	ARDS
Hypotension	Myocardial depression
	Liver failure
Tachycardia	Acute renal failure
	GI mucosal damage
'Cold, cyanosed' or 'Warm, flushed' peripheries	
Reduced urine output	DIC and haemorrhage 'purpura' 'Bleeding injection and line sites'
	Ischaemia Gangrene

(c) Clinical evaluation

Measure CVP (±PCWP)

	High >2		Low <2	
Warm or cold peripheries	Cold	Warm	Warm	Cold
Pulse volume	Low	High	High	Low
Diagnosis	Cardiogenic (MI) Obstructive (PE/pneumo-thorax) or Septic shock	Sepsis or CO₂ retention or Over transfusion	Sepsis or Anaphylaxis	Haemorrhage or Fluid loss or Anaphylaxis

Definition and causes

Shock is a loosely defined term. It describes the clinical syndrome that occurs when acute circulatory failure with inadequate or inappropriately distributed tissue perfusion results in failure to meet tissue metabolic demands causing generalized cellular hypoxia with or without lactic acidosis.

Shock can be classified into six categories.

1 Hypovolaemic: due to major reductions in circulating blood volume caused by haemorrhage, plasma loss (e.g. burns, pancreatitis) or extracellular fluid loss (e.g. diabetic ketoacidosis, trauma).

2 Cardiogenic: due to severe heart failure (e.g. myocardial infarction, acute mitral regurgitation).

3 Obstructive: caused by circulatory obstruction (e.g. pulmonary embolism, cardiac tamponade).

4 Septic: with infection or septicaemia (e.g. *Escherichia coli*). Vasodilation, arteriovenous shunting and capillary damage (Fig. a) cause subsequent hypotension and maldistribution of flow.

5 Anaphylactic: due to allergen-induced vasodilation (e.g. bee sting, peanut and other food allergies).

6 Neurogenic (spinal): follows high traumatic spinal cord lesions (above T_6). Interruption of sympathetic outflow causes vasodilation, hypothermia and bradycardia, which may be severe if vagal stimulation (e.g. pain, hypoxia) is unopposed.

Clinical features

Clinical features depend on the underlying cause (Chapters 20, 27, 44) and severity. General features include hypotension (systolic BP <100 mmHg), tachycardia (>100 beats/min), rapid respiration (>30/min), oliguria (urine output <30 mL/h) and drowsiness, confusion or agitation (Fig. b). Shock is either:

• **'cold, clammy' shock** (e.g. hypovolaemic, cardiogenic, obstructive, late septic) with cold peripheries (skin vasoconstriction), weak pulses and evidence of low cardiac output (e.g. oliguria, peripheral cyanosis, confusion); or

• **'warm, dilated' shock** (e.g. early septic, anaphylactic) with warm peripheries (skin vasodilation), bounding pulses and a high cardiac output (i.e. flushed).

Investigations

Investigations include routine blood tests, blood gases, lactic acid measurement, cardiac enzymes and blood cross-matching if haemorrhage is suspected. **Monitor vital signs:** temperature, respiratory rate, S_aO_2 and urine output. **Haemodynamic assessment** often requires intra-arterial BP measurement, CVP and ECG monitoring. Additional measurements (Chapter 2) are occasionally necessary (e.g. CO, SVR, PCWP, S_vO_2). **Radiology** includes chest radiographs. **Microbiology** requires examination of blood, sputum and urine samples.

Assessment

Clinical features, CVP and SVR define the cause of shock (Fig. c). Measurement of CVP, pulmonary capillary wedge pressure (PCWP) and SVR (Chapter 2) is useful when clinical signs are difficult to interpret. For example:

• CVP is: (i) **reduced** in hypovolaemic and anaphylactic shock; (ii) **elevated** in cardiogenic and obstructive shock; (iii) **low, normal or high** in septic shock.

• SVR is: (i) **high** in cardiogenic shock with sympathetic mediated vasoconstriction ($\rightarrow$ 'cold, clammy' patient) or (ii) **low** in septic vasodilation due to release of inflammatory mediators ($\rightarrow$ 'warm, dilated' patient).

Consequently, simple haemodynamic patterns may aid diagnosis.

• Hypovolaemic shock = low CVP/PCWP + CO + high SVR
• Cardiogenic shock = high CVP/PCWP + low CO + high SVR
• Septic shock = low CVP/PCWP + high CO + low SVR

Complications

Circulatory failure with tissue hypoxia results in multiorgan failure including acute respiratory distress syndrome (ARDS), systemic inflammatory response syndrome (SIRS), acute renal failure, and mucosal (e.g. peptic) ulceration (Figs a and b). A cycle of increasing 'oxygen debt' and 'shock-induced' tissue damage develops as decreased myocardial contractility and hypoxaemia (e.g. due to ARDS) further impair oxygen delivery and tissue oxygenation (Fig. a). Ischaemic damage to the intestinal mucosa causes bacterial and toxin translocation into the splanchnic circulation and further organ impairment. Eventually, 'refractory' shock develops with irreversible tissue damage and death.

Management

Early treatment is vital ('the golden hour'); mortality increases if shock lasts >1 h. Management aims to correct the underlying cause, reverse 'the tissue oxygen debt' and prevent the vicious cycle of progressive organ damage. Treatment of cardiogenic, obstructive, anaphylactic and septic shock is presented in later chapters. However, features common to the management of all forms of shock are:

1 Identify and treat the cause (e.g. sepsis)

2 Correct hypoxaemia with supplemental oxygen. In the absence of lung disease, severe shock will cause hypoxia due to reduced pulmonary blood flow, ventilation/perfusion (V/Q) mismatch and low S_vO_2. **Intubation and ventilation:** Indications for intubation (Chapter 9) include progressive hypoxaemia ($P_aO_2 < 8$ kPa on > 40% O_2), hypercapnia ($P_aCO_2 > 7.5$ kPa) or respiratory rate > 35/min. In obtunded patients, the high risk of aspiration necessitates a low threshold for intubation. Ventilatory support (Chapters 8, 10) reduces work of breathing, improves cardiac function and increases tissue oxygen delivery. Non-invasive ventilation (e.g. continuous positive airways pressure (CPAP)) may avoid the need for intubation.

3 Resuscitation requires appropriate **fluid management** (Chapter 5) and is critically dependent on the cause of shock and CVP ($\pm$ PCWP). For example, *hypovolaemia with low CVP/PCWP* requires fluid replacement, whereas *cardiogenic shock with raised CVP/PCWP* needs fluid restriction (although fluid administration may be required in right ventricular infarction!). The time course is also important. At the onset of septic shock fluid replacement is essential, but later, if ARDS develops, fluid restriction may be necessary to prevent pulmonary oedema (Chapter 26).

Inotropic support (Chapter 5) is indicated when *hypotension* (i.e. mean arterial pressure (MAP) <60 mmHg) or *tissue hypoxaemia* (e.g. oliguria) persists despite adequate fluid replacement or when fluid resuscitation is contraindicated (e.g. cardiogenic shock). The type of inotropic support will depend on the cause of shock. For example, **in septic shock** ('warm, dilated' patient), the CO is high but vasodilation and the associated low SVR may cause hypotension, inadequate tissue perfusion and organ hypoxia (e.g. oliguria, confusion). In this situation, noradrenaline, a peripheral vasoconstrictor, increases SVR, restoring blood pressure and tissue perfusion. **In cardiogenic shock** ('cold, clammy' patient), the CO is low due to poor myocardial contractility and SVR is high due to sympathetic vasoconstriction. Treatment with dobutamine increases myocardial contractility and reduces SVR.

Correction of severe acidosis with sodium bicarbonate is controversial but may be considered when pH is <7.1 with a normal P_aCO_2 (i.e. base excess > –8).

4 Remove circulatory obstructions. This includes: (i) thrombolysis for pulmonary embolism; (ii) drainage of cardiac tamponade/pneumothorax; and (iii) correction of DIC to prevent microcirculatory obstruction.

5 Circulatory support: fluids and inotropes

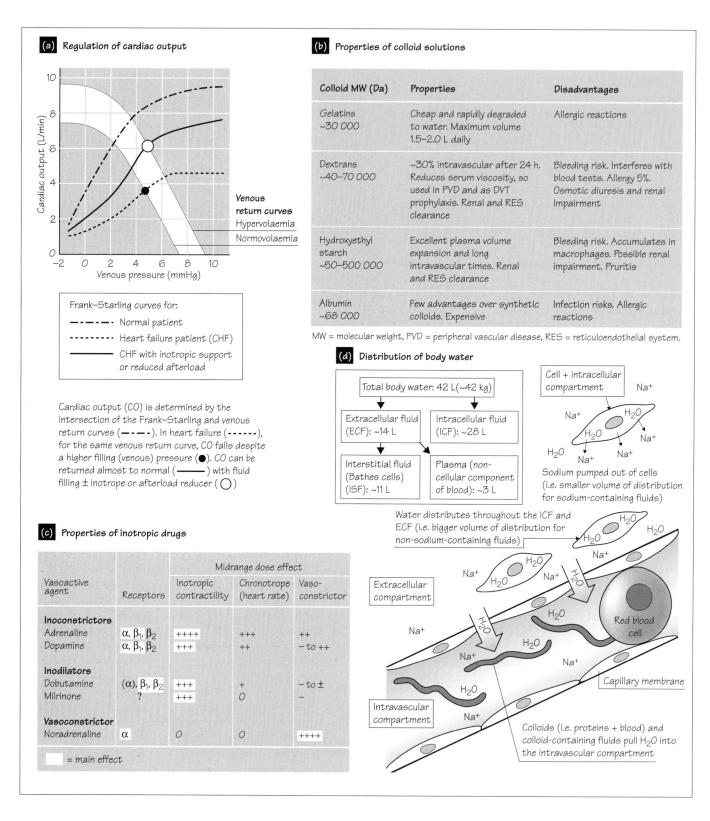

(a) Regulation of cardiac output

Frank–Starling curves for:
- — · — · — Normal patient
- · · · · · · Heart failure patient (CHF)
- ——— CHF with inotropic support or reduced afterload

Cardiac output (CO) is determined by the intersection of the Frank–Starling and venous return curves (— · — ·). In heart failure (· · · · · ·), for the same venous return curve, CO falls despite a higher filling (venous) pressure (●). CO can be returned almost to normal (———) with fluid filling ± inotrope or afterload reducer (○)

(b) Properties of colloid solutions

Colloid MW (Da)	Properties	Disadvantages
Gelatins ~30 000	Cheap and rapidly degraded to water. Maximum volume 1.5–2.0 L daily	Allergic reactions
Dextrans ~40–70 000	~30% intravascular after 24 h. Reduces serum viscosity, so used in PVD and as DVT prophylaxis. Renal and RES clearance	Bleeding risk. Interferes with blood tests. Allergy 5%. Osmotic diuresis and renal impairment
Hydroxyethyl starch ~50–500 000	Excellent plasma volume expansion and long intravascular times. Renal and RES clearance	Bleeding risk. Accumulates in macrophages. Possible renal impairment. Pruritis
Albumin ~68 000	Few advantages over synthetic colloids. Expensive	Infection risks. Allergic reactions

MW = molecular weight, PVD = peripheral vascular disease, RES = reticuloendothelial system.

(d) Distribution of body water

Total body water: 42 L (~42 kg)

Extracellular fluid (ECF): ~14 L

Intracellular fluid (ICF): ~28 L

Interstitial fluid (Bathes cells) (ISF): ~11 L

Plasma (non-cellular component of blood): ~3 L

Cell + intracellular compartment

Sodium pumped out of cells (i.e. smaller volume of distribution for sodium-containing fluids)

Water distributes throughout the ICF and ECF (i.e. bigger volume of distribution for non-sodium-containing fluids)

Extracellular compartment

Intravascular compartment

Red blood cell

Capillary membrane

Colloids (i.e. proteins + blood) and colloid-containing fluids pull H_2O into the intravascular compartment

(c) Properties of inotropic drugs

Vasoactive agent	Receptors	Midrange dose effect		
		Inotropic contractility	Chronotrope (heart rate)	Vaso-constrictor
Inoconstrictors				
Adrenaline	α, β₁, β₂	++++	+++	++
Dopamine	α, β₁, β₂	+++	++	– to ++
Inodilators				
Dobutamine	(α), β₁, β₂	+++	+	– to ±
Milrinone	?	+++	0	–
Vasoconstrictor				
Noradrenaline	α	0	0	++++

□ = main effect

Circulatory failure or **shock** (Chapter 4) occurs when cardiac output (CO) and/or blood pressure (BP) are inadequate to maintain tissue blood supply and meet metabolic requirements. **Causes** include heart failure, hypovolaemia, circulatory obstruction and inappropriate vasodilation (e.g. sepsis).

Circulatory assessment must address:
- **Cardiac function** to evaluate CO and exclude heart failure (Chapter 20). CO is the product of **stroke volume (SV)** and **heart rate (HR)**, where SV is dependent on:

  (i) **preload** — a function of ventricular end-diastolic volume and thus venous return and pressure (Fig. a);

  (ii) **afterload** — the load against which the ventricle has to work. Aortic stenosis, high SVR, negative intrathoracic pressure and left ventricular (LV) dilation increase LV afterload;

  (iii) **myocardial contractility** — the heart's ability to perform work independently of pre- or afterload.

Clinical assessment of CO in terms of pulse volume, HR, BP, CVP and peripheral perfusion is often adequate (Chapter 4) but direct measurements (Chapter 2) may be required to optimize circulatory performance in critical illness.
- **Circuit factors** (e.g. hypovolaemia, obstruction, vasodilation) including venous filling pressures (e.g. CVP, PCWP), BP, SVR and tissue hypoxia (Chapters 2, 4).

Circulatory support involves a hierarchy of management.

1 *Diagnosis* determines treatment (e.g. fluid restriction in left heart failure vs. fluid resuscitation in hypovolaemia). Monitoring, supplemental oxygen and temperature control are essential. Antibiotics are required for infection, thrombolysis for myocardial infarction and analgesia for pain-induced vasovagal hypotension.

2 *Rate and rhythm.* Both tachycardia (e.g. arrhythmias) and bradycardia (e.g. vagal tone) can reduce CO. Restoring sinus rhythm and a normal HR improve BP and CO. Initially electrolyte concentrations ($K^+ > 4.5$ mmol/L, $Mg^{2+} > 1.4$ mmol/L) are optimized and arrhythmogenic drugs (e.g. salbutamol) withdrawn. Antiarrhythmic drugs or cardioversion may be required depending on haemodynamic stability (Chapters 19, 21).

3 *Fluid therapy* aims to optimize preload (Fig. a). The response to a **'fluid challenge'** (~250 mL over <20 min) often determines the need for volume replacement (Chapter 2). A sustained increase in filling pressures (CVP, PCWP) with little or no increase in CO indicates that the heart is operating on the flat part of the Starling curve (Fig. a). Further fluid administration risks pulmonary oedema (Chapter 20). A transient increase in filling pressures, CO and BP suggests the need for further fluid. Selection of appropriate fluid for replacement (crystalloid vs. colloid) is controversial. In general, crystalloid solutions are used first, or the fluid that is lost is replaced (e.g. blood during haemorrhage). Specific fluid properties can also be utilized.
- **Crystalloid solutions** are water to which solutes (e.g. sodium chloride, glucose) have been added. Although inexpensive and usually isotonic, they redistribute rapidly (~1–4 h; Fig. d). Low-sodium fluids like 5% dextrose disperse throughout the intracellular and extracellular fluid (ICF, ECF), whereas sodium-containing fluids like normal saline (NS) only disseminate into the ECF as cell membrane pumps remove sodium from the ICF. Consequently, NS is preferred for volume expansion as it has a smaller volume of distribution. Nevertheless, large volumes of crystalloid are required to replace plasma loss, which may cause oedema.
- **Colloid solutions** contain large molecules that cannot easily diffuse out of blood vessels. They exert an oncotic pressure which pulls water into, and may expand, the intravascular compartment. Although expensive, colloids remain intravascular for long periods and ~4 times as much crystalloid is required to achieve the same volume expansion. Consequently, colloids are used when crystalloid infusions cannot maintain adequate intravascular filling or when excessive fluid is contraindicated (e.g. pulmonary oedema). Natural colloids are blood and albumin. Synthetic colloids include gelatin, dextran and hydroxyethyl starch. Disadvantages include allergic reactions, clotting abnormalities and renal impairment (Table b).
- **Blood** is usually given to maintain Hb concentration >80 g/L (>8 g/dL). However, young patients and those with renal disease or chronic anaemia may tolerate lower levels. In cardiac patients an Hb ~100 g/L (~10 g/dL) improves outcome.

4 *Inotropic and vasoactive drugs* provide further haemodynamic support when optimal HR and preload fail to correct circulatory failure. Inotropes are usually administered through central lines, responses monitored and therapy titrated to specific endpoints (e.g. MAP 65–70 mmHg). Hypovolaemia, acidosis (pH < 7.1) and electrolyte derangement (e.g. hypokalaemia) impair inotropic drug actions and should be corrected to ensure maximal effect. In volume-replete patients, appropriate inotropic therapy depends on the cause of circulatory failure (e.g. vasodilation) and drug receptor properties (Table c). Activation of α **receptors** causes peripheral vasoconstriction, β_1 **receptors** are chronotropic ($\uparrow$ HR) and inotropic and β_2 **receptors** cause vasodilation and bronchodilation. A drug may activate several receptors (e.g. adrenaline (epinephrine) has α, β_1, β_2 properties), but the balance varies (e.g. dobutamine also has α, β_1, β_2 properties but β_1, β_2 effects are greater than α properties). Initially a single drug is selected but the correct balance of receptor stimulation may require drug combinations. For example:
- **In septic shock** profound vasodilation causes hypotension despite a high CO. Initially noradrenaline (norepinephrine), an α vasoconstrictor, maintains BP and organ perfusion. However, prolonged sepsis may impair cardiac contractility requiring a β_1 inotropic agent to maintain CO (e.g. dobutamine).
- **In myocardial ischaemia** dobutamine β_1 properties increase cardiac contractility without raising myocardial oxygen consumption, whilst β_2 vasodilator properties reduce afterload and increase CO. However, noradrenaline (epinephrine)-mediated α vasoconstriction may be required to offset hypotension induced by high-dose dobutamine β_2 vasodilation.

The concept that drug concentration determines receptor stimulation is controversial. In particular, there is little evidence that low-concentration dopamine increases renal blood flow by stimulating dopaminergic receptors, whilst high concentrations stimulate α and β receptors.

5 *Other methods of circulatory support* are occasionally required. **Cardiac pacemakers** increase CO (Chapter 19) and **ventilatory support** reduces cardiorespiratory work and pulmonary oedema (Chapters 8, 10).

Intra-aortic balloon pumps are valuable in IHD, ventricular septal defect (VSD) and whilst awaiting heart transplantation. They are sited in the descending aorta above the renal arteries. Diastolic balloon inflation enhances coronary and systemic perfusion pressures whilst systolic deflation increases CO by reducing afterload. Complications include renal and mesenteric ischaemia, infection and aortic dissection.

Left ventricular assist devices are currently being developed.

6 Oxygenation failure and oxygen therapy

(a) Relationship between oxygen tension (PO_2) and haemoglobin saturation (SO_2)

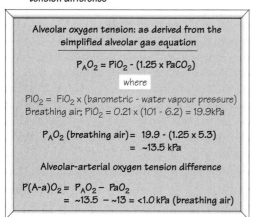

y-axis: Haemoglobin saturation (SO_2%) — 0, 20, 40, 60, 80, 100
x-axis: PO_2 (mmHg) — 0, 20, 40, 60, 80, 100

P_{50}

↑ Temperature
↑ $PaCO_2$ (Bohr effect)
↓ pH / metabolic acidosis
↑ 2,3 DPG

(b) Alveolar oxygen tension and alveolar-arterial oxygen tension difference

Alveolar oxygen tension: as derived from the simplified alveolar gas equation

$$P_AO_2 = PiO_2 - (1.25 \times PaCO_2)$$

where

$PiO_2 = FiO_2 \times$ (barometric - water vapour pressure)
Breathing air; $PiO_2 = 0.21 \times (101 - 6.2) = 19.9$ kPa

$$P_AO_2 \text{ (breathing air)} = 19.9 - (1.25 \times 5.3)$$
$$= \sim13.5 \text{ kPa}$$

Alveolar-arterial oxygen tension difference

$$P(A\text{-}a)O_2 = P_AO_2 - PaO_2$$
$$= \sim13.5 - \sim13 = <1.0 \text{ kPa (breathing air)}$$

P_AO_2 = alveolar oxygen tension, PiO_2 = inspired oxygen tension,
FiO_2 = fractional concentration of oxygen in inspired air,
$P(A\text{-}a)O_2$ = alveolar-arterial oxygen tension difference,
PaO_2 = arterial oxygen tension, $PaCO_2$ = arterial CO_2 tension

(c) Simple oxygen delivery systems

High-flow (Venturi) face-mask (~24–40% O_2)
- The O_2 flow through the jet mixing Venturi valve entrains the correct proportion of air to produce the required O_2 concentration (i.e. 24%)
- More gas is delivered than is required by the patient (i.e. 30 L/min)
- Consequently the inspired O_2 concentration is unaffected by the patient's breathing pattern
- Used in COPD with respiratory failure to avoid CO_2 retention

30 L/min total gas flow at fixed O_2 concentration
2 L/min jet of oxygen
25 L/min escapes from mask
14 L/min entrained air
30 L/min into mask at FiO_2 24%
5 L/min inspired

Low-flow mask (~30–60% O_2)
- Oxygen flows at a set rate into the mask and is supplemented by air drawn into the mask
- FiO_2 achieved depends on ventilation
  i.e. Ventilation = 5 L/min
  O_2 flow = 2 L/min; air flow (21% O_2) = 3 L/min
  $FiO_2 = (2 + 0.21 \times 3)/5 \times 100 = 53\%$
  i.e. Ventilation = 25 L/min
  O_2 flow = 2 L/min; air flow (21% O_2) = 23 L/min
  $FiO_2 = (2 + 0.21 \times 23)/25 \times 100 = 27\%$
- Not recommended when accurate control of FiO_2 desirable, e.g. COPD with hypercapnia

3 L/min air drawn into mask
2 L/min oxygen into mask
5 L/min inspired
2 L/min oxygen

Non-rebreathing and anaesthetic masks (>60% O_2)
- Deliver high oxygen concentrations (i.e. FiO_2 >60%) (see Chapters 7, 9)
- Non-rebreathing masks have a reservoir which increases the inspired oxygen concentration by preventing oxygen loss during expiration

Nasal prongs
- Deliver a constant O_2 flow, therefore FiO_2 varies with ventilation
- More comfortable than a mask
- No need to remove during eating or expectoration
- O_2 delivered by nose is inhaled even during mouth breathing

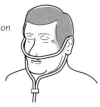

(d) Effect of true shunt (Q_S/Q_T) and ventilation/perfusion mismatch on the arterial oxygen tension (PaO_2) and inspired oxygen fraction (FiO_2) relationship

True shunt
Shunt fraction = Q_S/Q_T (%)
10%
30%
50%
FiO_2 — 0.2, 1.0

Hypoxaemia caused by true right to left shunt is refractory to supplemental O_2 when 'shunt fraction' exceeds 30%

Ventilation/perfusion (V/Q) mismatch
PaO_2 (kPa) — 70.0, 14, 7
A
B
FiO_2 — 0.2, 1.0

Reductions in PaO_2 caused by V/Q mismatch respond to O_2 but the response depends on whether there are many units with mild V/Q mismatch (A) or a few units with very low V/Q ratios (B)

(e) Risks associated with high-dose oxygen therapy

1. **Carbon dioxide retention:**
   ~10% of breathless patients, mainly COPD, have type II respiratory failure (RF)
   ~40-50% of COPD patients are at risk of type II RF
2. **Absorption collapse**
   O_2 in poorly ventilated alveoli is rapidly absorbed causing collapse; whereas N_2 absorption is slow
3. **Pulmonary oxygen toxicity**
   FiO_2>60% may damage alveolar membranes causing ARDS if inhaled for >24-48h (Chapter 26)
4. **Fire**
   Deaths and burns occur when patients smoke during O_2 therapy
5. **Paul-Bert effect**
   Breathing hyperbaric O_2 can cause cerebral vasoconstriction and epileptic fits

Respiratory failure

Respiratory failure (RF) is due to inadequate gas exchange.

- **Type I RF (oxygenation failure)** occurs when blood bypasses or is not fully oxygenated in the lungs causing **hypoxaemia** (low P_aO_2). P_aCO_2 is normal or low because ventilation is unchanged or increased due to breathlessness. **Causes** include V/Q mismatch, right to left shunts and low inspired O_2 (e.g. high altitude). Oxygenation is improved by re-expansion of collapsed alveoli, O_2 therapy and reducing V/Q mismatch (Chapters 8, 10).
- **Type II RF (ventilatory failure).** Hypoventilation reduces CO_2 clearance causing **hypercapnia** (high P_aCO_2) *with or without hypoxaemia*. **Causes** include respiratory muscle weakness, chest wall deformity (e.g. kyphoscoliosis), impaired respiratory drive (e.g. opioid overdose) and excessive work of breathing (WoB). In critical illness, the WoB required to ventilate abnormal lungs may be >30% of total O_2 consumption (normally < 5%). Ventilation is improved and WoB reduced by decreasing airways resistance (e.g. bronchodilation), ventilatory support (Chapters 8, 10) and better compliance (e.g. secretion clearance, alveolar recruitment).

Tissue hypoxia

Tissue hypoxia occurs within 4 min of cardiorespiratory arrest as O_2 reserves are small. **Causes** (Chapter 3) include: (i) **hypoxaemia** secondary to RF; (ii) **failure of oxygen transport** due to reduced blood flow, anaemia or haemoglobinopathy; and (iii) **failure of tissue oxygen utilization** during sepsis or poisoning (e.g. cyanide). Successful therapy requires early recognition but **clinical features** are often non-specific including altered mental state, dyspnoea, hyperventilation, arrhythmias and hypotension. **Central cyanosis** is detected when reduced Hb is > 1.5–5 g/dL. It is a poor indicator of hypoxia as it may be absent in hypoxic, anaemic patients but apparent in normoxic, polycythaemic subjects.

Monitoring oxygenation (Chapter 2)

Saturation of Hb with O_2 (SO_2) is determined by the partial pressure of O_2 (PO_2) in blood. The oxyhaemoglobin curve describes this relationship (Fig. a). **Arterial PO_2** (P_aO_2) is the tension driving O_2 into the tissues, and **arterial SO_2** (S_aO_2) reflects the level of O_2 carriage by Hb molecules. **Pulse oximetry** and **blood gas analysis** measure S_aO_2 and P_aO_2, respectively. These are the principal measures used to initiate, monitor and adjust O_2 therapy. However, they can be normal when tissue hypoxia is caused by low cardiac output, anaemia or failure of O_2 utilization. In these circumstances, **mixed venous oxygen saturation** (S_vO_2) < 55–60% (normally > 70%) may indicate inadequate tissue O_2 supply (Chapter 2). P_aO_2/F_iO_2 **ratio** is a convenient index of O_2 exchange that adjusts for inspired O_2 concentration (F_iO_2). **Alveolar–arterial oxygen tension difference** ($P_{(A-a)}O_2$) also determines efficiency of gas exchange. P_AO_2 is calculated from the simplified alveolar gas equation (Fig. b). By incorporating CO_2 tension it eliminates hypoventilation and hypercapnia as the main causes of hypoxaemia. Detection of **single-organ ischaemia** is difficult, involving techniques with significant limitations (e.g. gastric tonometry).

Acute oxygen therapy

The main indications for instituting O_2 therapy are **cardiorespiratory arrest**, **hypoxaemia** (P_aO_2 < 8 kPa, S_aO_2 < 90%), **hypotension**, **low cardiac output**, **metabolic acidosis** and **respiratory distress**. Emergency O_2 therapy should be delivered by facemask, and early arterial blood gas (ABG) assessment is essential. The important features of different oxygen delivery systems are illustrated in Fig. (c). Nasal prongs are best used in stable patients.

Oxygen dosage

Inadequate O_2 therapy causes more deaths and disability than can be justified by the risks associated with high-dose O_2 (Fig. e). In particular, type II RF only affects ~10% of breathless patients, most of whom have chronic obstructive pulmonary disease (COPD) with reduced respiratory drive. In these patients, O_2 therapy can precipitate or aggravate hypercapnia and respiratory acidosis. Consequently, appropriate O_2 administration is difficult in early (prediagnostic) critical illness:

- **Before blood gas measurement** the risk of hypoxia is usually greater than that of hypercapnia. During the short period (<20 min) of prehospital transport and emergency department assessment, continuous O_2 therapy (Fig. c) should maintain S_aO_2 >90%. This is usually achieved with ~40–60% O_2 via a medium concentration facemask. Following major trauma, severe haemorrhage, cardiorespiratory arrest, overdose and carbon monoxide poisoning, or in severely hypoxic patients, high-dose O_2 (60–100%) is administered through a reservoir, non-rebreathing mask. If COPD or type II RF is suspected, initial O_2 therapy (~40%) is titrated to maintain S_aO_2 at ~90–93%. Controlled O_2 therapy using a fixed performance (24–35%) Venturi mask is preferable if drowsiness develops or if type II RF has occurred previously.
- **After blood gas measurement** non-COPD patients (e.g. pneumonia, trauma) continue with medium or high concentration O_2 therapy as described above. In COPD, with or without initial hypercapnia, O_2 therapy is best given via a Venturi mask and is titrated to the lowest concentration required to achieve S_aO_2 90–93% (P_aO_2 8 kPa). Higher S_aO_2 has no advantages but may cause or exacerbate hypercapnia and respiratory acidosis. ABGs must be monitored regularly. If P_aCO_2 rises (> 10.5 kPa), pH falls (< 7.25), or if the patient becomes drowsy or fatigued, non-invasive ventilation (NIV) should be initiated (Chapter 8). Earlier NIV (i.e. pH < 7.35) is beneficial in some cases. If hypercapnia and respiratory acidosis progress but intubation and mechanical ventilation are considered inappropriate (i.e. end-stage disease), F_iO_2 is reduced to stimulate hypoxic drive and spontaneous ventilation, thereby decreasing P_aCO_2. S_aO_2 will fall to < 90%, but aim to maintain P_aO_2 at > 6.5 kPa. Nebulizers should be driven with compressed air in hypercapnic patients.

Efficacy of oxygen therapy

- **Hypoxaemic patients** benefit most. Figure (d) illustrates the effect of F_iO_2 on P_aO_2 in patients with right to left shunts and V/Q mismatch. A true shunt >30% causes persistent hypoxaemia despite increased F_iO_2. Improved oxygenation requires reduction of shunt (e.g. recruitment of collapsed alveoli) and V/Q mismatch (Chapters 8, 10). In alveolar hypoventilation (e.g. opiate overdose), O_2, therapy relieves hypoxaemia but only improved ventilation (e.g. NIV) corrects hypercapnia (Chapter 8).
- **Patients without hypoxaemia** benefit less. In **low-output cardiac states**, high F_iO_2 only marginally improves oxygenation because Hb is fully saturated and O_2 solubility is low. These patients require early restoration of tissue blood flow. In **carbon monoxide poisoning**, high-dose O_2 is essential, despite a normal P_aO_2, to reduce carboxyhaemoglobin half-life (Chapter 49).

7 Airways management

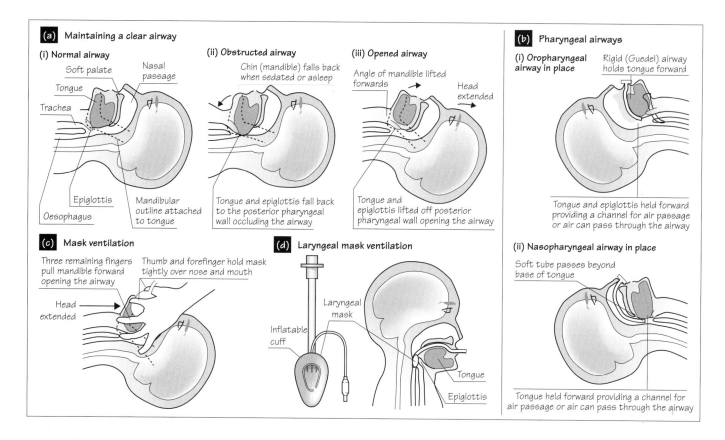

(a) Maintaining a clear airway

(i) Normal airway
- Soft palate
- Nasal passage
- Tongue
- Trachea
- Epiglottis
- Oesophagus
- Mandibular outline attached to tongue

(ii) Obstructed airway
- Chin (mandible) falls back when sedated or asleep
- Tongue and epiglottis fall back to the posterior pharyngeal wall occluding the airway

(iii) Opened airway
- Angle of mandible lifted forwards
- Head extended
- Tongue and epiglottis lifted off posterior pharyngeal wall opening the airway

(b) Pharyngeal airways

(i) Oropharyngeal airway in place
- Rigid (Guedel) airway holds tongue forward
- Tongue and epiglottis held forward providing a channel for air passage or air can pass through the airway

(ii) Nasopharyngeal airway in place
- Soft tube passes beyond base of tongue
- Tongue held forward providing a channel for air passage or air can pass through the airway

(c) Mask ventilation
- Three remaining fingers pull mandible forward opening the airway
- Thumb and forefinger hold mask tightly over nose and mouth
- Head extended

(d) Laryngeal mask ventilation
- Laryngeal mask
- Inflatable cuff
- Tongue
- Epiglottis

Airways obstruction is a life-threatening emergency and is particularly perilous when cardiorespiratory function is compromised. All critical care staff must be able to establish a patent airway and restore adequate ventilation.

Oropharyngeal obstruction is usually caused by the tongue (Fig. a) but may be due to foreign bodies, tumours or laryngospasm.

Complete obstruction is characterized by absent airflow, no breath sounds and chest wall intercostal recession.

Partial obstruction reduces airflow despite increased respiratory effort and may be accompanied by laryngeal 'stridor' or nasopharyngeal 'snoring'.

Airways management

- **Clear the airway** of secretions and remove foreign bodies. Upper airways obstruction is often due to occlusion of the posterior pharyngeal space by the tongue (in obtunded or sedated patients) (Fig. a(i, ii)). Lifting the mandible forward and slightly extending the neck (jaw lift) can often restore airflow (Fig. a(iii)).
- **Oropharyngeal airways** establish an airway when jaw lift is inadequate. They are useful during mask ventilation (see below), particularly in edentulous patients.

  Rigid oropharyngeal (Guedel) airways lift the tongue and epiglottis away from the posterior pharyngeal wall (Fig. b(i)). The airway is inserted upside down and rotated 180° into position. Care is required to avoid damaging the teeth or pushing the tongue backwards and increasing obstruction. Guedel airways are only used in obtunded patients as they provoke gag reflexes, vomiting and laryngospasm in conscious patients.

  Soft nasopharyngeal airways (SNPAs) can be used in alert patients. They extend beyond the base of the tongue to create an air passage (Fig. b(ii)). Topical nasal anaesthesia and lubrication (e.g. lidocaine gel) reduce insertion discomfort but traumatic epistaxis may occur. Contraindications to SNPAs include coagulopathy, nasal obstruction and basilar skull fractures.
- **Mask ventilation** allows ventilatory support in non-intubated patients. In conjunction with jaw lift the increased oropharyngeal pressure during ventilation alleviates airways obstruction.

  Anaesthetic facemasks are available in a variety of shapes and sizes to ensure a tight fit. Firm downward pressure on the mask with the thumb and forefinger maintains a seal whilst the mandible is simultaneously lifted with the three remaining fingers and the head extended to optimize the airway during ventilation (Fig. c). A two-handed technique with an assistant to squeeze the bag may be required. Unfortunately, mask ventilation may be impossible in some patients.
- **Laryngeal mask airways** are useful when intubation fails. They sit over the laryngeal inlet allowing temporary ventilation in sedated or obtunded patients (Fig. d). Potential problems (e.g. laryngospasm, aspiration) limit use in ICU.
- **Endotracheal intubation** (Chapter 9) may be required if adequate ventilation cannot be achieved. Occasionally an **emergency cricothyroidotomy** is required to establish a direct tracheal airway (Chapters 11, 29).

8 Non-invasive ventilation

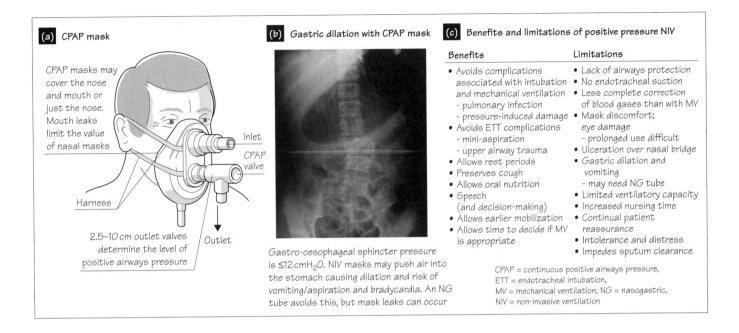

(a) CPAP mask

CPAP masks may cover the nose and mouth or just the nose. Mouth leaks limit the value of nasal masks

Inlet

CPAP valve

Harness

Outlet

2.5–10 cm outlet valves determine the level of positive airways pressure

(b) Gastric dilation with CPAP mask

Gastro-oesophageal sphincter pressure is ≤12 cmH₂O. NIV masks may push air into the stomach causing dilation and risk of vomiting/aspiration and bradycardia. An NG tube avoids this, but mask leaks can occur

(c) Benefits and limitations of positive pressure NIV

Benefits	Limitations

• Avoids complications associated with intubation and mechanical ventilation
  - pulmonary infection
  - pressure-induced damage
• Avoids ETT complications
  - mini-aspiration
  - upper airway trauma
• Allows rest periods
• Preserves cough
• Allows oral nutrition
• Speech
  (and decision-making)
• Allows earlier mobilization
• Allows time to decide if MV is appropriate
	• Lack of airways protection
	• No endotracheal suction
	• Less complete correction of blood gases than with MV
	• Mask discomfort; eye damage
	  - prolonged use difficult
	• Ulceration over nasal bridge
	• Gastric dilation and vomiting
	  - may need NG tube
	• Limited ventilatory capacity
	• Increased nursing time
	• Continual patient reassurance
	• Intolerance and distress
	• Impedes sputum clearance

CPAP = continuous positive airways pressure,
ETT = endotracheal intubation,
MV = mechanical ventilation, NG = nasogastric,
NIV = non-invasive ventilation

Non-invasive ventilation (NIV) is provided by machines that support ventilation and assist gas exchange without the need for endotracheal intubation (ETI). It is most successful in alert, cooperative, self-ventilating, haemodynamically stable patients who are able to protect and clear their airways.

Indications include respiratory support during acute (e.g. COPD exacerbation) or chronic (e.g. neuromuscular disease) respiratory failure, when ETI is considered inappropriate (e.g. end-stage respiratory disease) and to aid weaning from mechanical ventilation.

Individual NIV techniques deliver varying degrees of ventilatory support and/or alveolar recruitment with corresponding reductions in WoB and/or improvements in oxygenation (Chapter 6).

1 Negative pressure ventilation (NPV) was originally developed to support victims of poliomyelitis-induced respiratory paralysis. Patients were placed in **tank ventilators** sealed at the neck. Lowering tank pressures expanded the chest causing inspiration. Expiration was passive. However, these 'iron lungs' were limited by difficulties with nursing access, poor CO₂ clearance and secretion retention which caused airways obstruction or pneumonia. NPV has largely been superseded by the development of positive pressure ventilators, which are particularly successful in the management of acute respiratory failure. NPV is now rarely used except in patients with chronic hypoventilation (e.g. kyphoscoliosis) or as part of rehabilitation programmes (e.g. spinal injury). Current NPV techniques include (i) **jacket (cuirass) ventilators,** which only produce a negative pressure around the chest but leaks often limit effectiveness, and (ii) **rocking beds,** which utilize gravity to enhance diaphragmatic movement.

2 Positive pressure NIV is delivered through tight-fitting nasal or full facemasks (Fig. a). Figure (c) lists potential benefits and disadvantages.

• **Nasal intermittent positive pressure ventilation** (NIPPV) delivers inspiratory pressure support (PS; ~10–30 cmH₂O), for a prescribed inspiratory time, adjusted according to the patient's requirements. It augments tidal volume (V_T), clears CO₂ and reduces WoB. Modern NIV ventilators also provide adjustable positive end-expiratory pressure (PEEP; Chapter 10). NIPPV is effective in chronic respiratory failure, primary alveolar hypoventilation, nocturnal hypoventilation and in some patients with acute exacerbations of COPD or acute hypercapnic respiratory failure who are tiring and cannot maintain WoB. Successful use requires well-trained staff, gradual introduction to a co-operative patient and careful synchronization of breathing with the ventilator.

• **Continuous positive airways pressure (CPAP).** Typically ~5–10 cmH₂O is maintained throughout inspiration and expiration by a flow generator. Resulting alveolar recruitment due to re-inflation of collapsed or oedematous lung reduces V/Q mismatch and improves oxygenation. Increased functional residual capacity (FRC) reduces WoB by moving the lung pressure–volume relationship into the steep part of the curve, making the lungs easier to inflate (i.e. increased compliance). CPAP is most successful when initiated early in diseases that respond to modest airways pressures (e.g. cardiogenic pulmonary oedema, pneumonia). It also helps prevent upper airways collapse in obstructive sleep apnoea. Both CPAP and PEEP may aid ventilation or weaning of COPD or asthma patients who are intubated or have tracheostomies by preventing small airways collapse and reducing gas trapping (Chapters 24, 25). A nasogastric tube prevents gastric distension and reduces the risk of aspiration (Fig. b).

• **Bilevel positive pressure ventilation** (BIPAP) delivers two levels of CPAP whilst allowing spontaneous respiration. The higher pressure augments alveolar ventilation and CO₂ clearance; the lower pressure maintains alveolar recruitment (Chapters 6, 10).

9 Endotracheal intubation

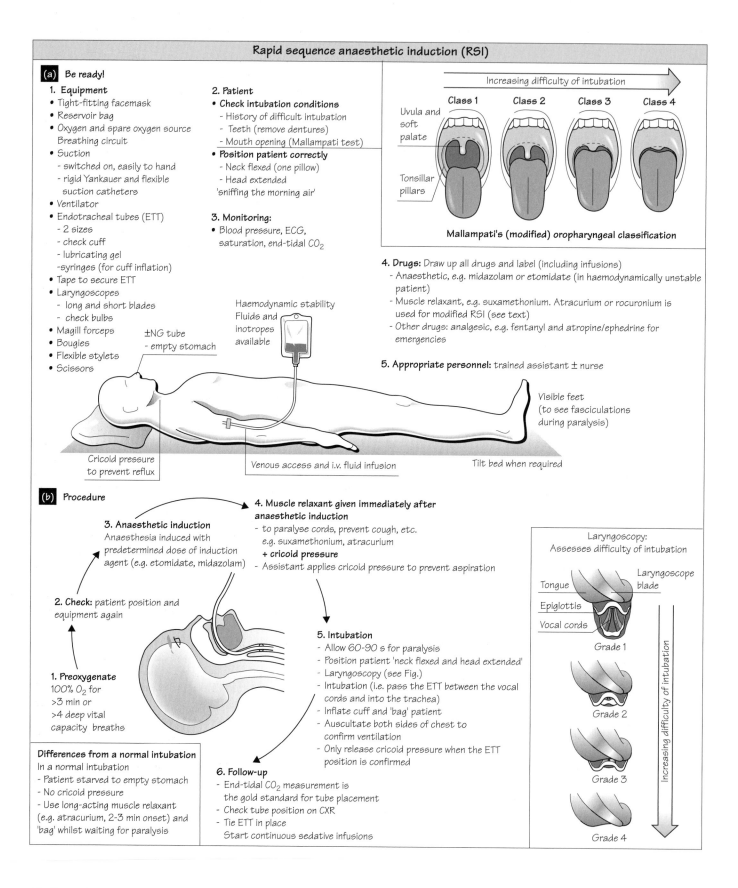

Rapid sequence anaesthetic induction (RSI)

(a) Be ready!

1. Equipment
- Tight-fitting facemask
- Reservoir bag
- Oxygen and spare oxygen source
  Breathing circuit
- Suction
  - switched on, easily to hand
  - rigid Yankauer and flexible
    suction catheters
- Ventilator
- Endotracheal tubes (ETT)
  - 2 sizes
  - check cuff
  - lubricating gel
  - syringes (for cuff inflation)
- Tape to secure ETT
- Laryngoscopes
  - long and short blades
  - check bulbs
- Magill forceps
- Bougies
- Flexible stylets
- Scissors

2. Patient
- **Check intubation conditions**
  - History of difficult intubation
  - Teeth (remove dentures)
  - Mouth opening (Mallampati test)
- **Position patient correctly**
  - Neck flexed (one pillow)
  - Head extended
  'sniffing the morning air'

3. Monitoring:
- Blood pressure, ECG,
  saturation, end-tidal CO_2

Mallampati's (modified) oropharyngeal classification

Increasing difficulty of intubation

Class 1   Class 2   Class 3   Class 4

Uvula and soft palate

Tonsillar pillars

4. Drugs: Draw up all drugs and label (including infusions)
- Anaesthetic, e.g. midazolam or etomidate (in haemodynamically unstable patient)
- Muscle relaxant, e.g. suxamethonium. Atracurium or rocuronium is used for modified RSI (see text)
- Other drugs: analgesic, e.g. fentanyl and atropine/ephedrine for emergencies

5. Appropriate personnel: trained assistant ± nurse

±NG tube
- empty stomach

Haemodynamic stability
Fluids and inotropes available

Visible feet
(to see fasciculations during paralysis)

Cricoid pressure to prevent reflux

Venous access and i.v. fluid infusion

Tilt bed when required

(b) Procedure

3. Anaesthetic induction
Anaesthesia induced with predetermined dose of induction agent (e.g. etomidate, midazolam)

4. Muscle relaxant given immediately after anaesthetic induction
- to paralyse cords, prevent cough, etc.
  e.g. suxamethonium, atracurium
  + cricoid pressure
- Assistant applies cricoid pressure to prevent aspiration

2. Check: patient position and equipment again

1. Preoxygenate
100% O_2 for
>3 min or
>4 deep vital capacity breaths

5. Intubation
- Allow 60-90 s for paralysis
- Position patient 'neck flexed and head extended'
- Laryngoscopy (see Fig.)
- Intubation (i.e. pass the ETT between the vocal cords and into the trachea)
- Inflate cuff and 'bag' patient
- Auscultate both sides of chest to confirm ventilation
- Only release cricoid pressure when the ETT position is confirmed

6. Follow-up
- End-tidal CO_2 measurement is the gold standard for tube placement
- Check tube position on CXR
- Tie ETT in place
  Start continuous sedative infusions

Differences from a normal intubation
In a normal intubation
- Patient starved to empty stomach
- No cricoid pressure
- Use long-acting muscle relaxant
  (e.g. atracurium, 2-3 min onset) and
  'bag' whilst waiting for paralysis

Laryngoscopy:
Assesses difficulty of intubation

Tongue
Epiglottis
Vocal cords

Laryngoscope blade

Grade 1

Grade 2

Grade 3

Grade 4

Increasing difficulty of intubation

Most intubations in critically ill patients are emergency procedures rendered particularly hazardous by haemodynamic instability, hypovolaemia, hypoxaemia, coexisting disease and potential aspiration of stomach contents. Whenever possible, appropriately trained clinicians skilled in airways management should perform ETI. However, during emergencies all critical care team members must be familiar with basic airways management (Chapter 7), ETI techniques and the failed intubation drill.

- **Indications for ETI** include respiratory failure (Chapter 6); airways protection from gastric aspiration; decreased level of consciousness (Glasgow Coma Score ≤8); secretion clearance; upper airways obstruction; raised intracranial pressure treatment; and surgical procedures.

- **Objective measures** suggesting the need for ventilatory support and ETI (if non-invasive ventilation is not possible) include a respiratory rate >35/min; vital capacity <15 mL/kg; $P_aO_2 < 8$ kPa on >40% O_2; $P_aCO_2 > 7.5$ kPa (except in chronic retainers); and occasionally alveolar–arterial (A–a) gradient >45 kPa on 100% O_2.

- **Airways assessment** only predicts ~50% of difficult ETIs (incidence ~1:65). **History:** When feasible, review anaesthetic notes and ask about previous difficult ETIs. **General examination** assesses cardiorespiratory status including oxygen therapy requirements. Patients with obesity, short necks or distorted neck anatomy (e.g. goitres) often present problems. **Airway examination** evaluates features associated with difficult ETI including: (i) absence of key anatomical landmarks during oropharyngeal inspection with tongue protrusion (e.g. faucial pillars, soft palate, uvula), as described in Mallampati's modified classification (Fig. a); (ii) short thyromental distance (i.e. < three fingerbreadths or 6 cm from thyroid cartilage to chin); (iii) restricted mouth opening (i.e. <4 cm); (iv) reduced neck extension; (v) oral factors (e.g. large tongue, buck teeth).

- **Routes of intubation.** Oral endotracheal tubes are usually preferred. They are relatively wide which reduces airways resistance and improves secretion clearance. Nasotracheal tubes are infrequently used (e.g. after oral trauma), but may improve comfort and oral hygiene. Disadvantages include high airways resistance (i.e. long, narrow tube), traumatic epistaxis and frequent sinusitis. They are contraindicated in nasal obstruction, sinusitis or base of skull fractures.

- **Preparation for intubation.** All equipment must be immediately available (Fig. a). Intravenous access should be established, but in critically ill patients clinical circumstances rarely permit full resuscitation, electrolyte correction or treatment of pre-existing conditions before ETI. **Preoxygenation** is always essential using tight-fitting facemasks to deliver 100% O_2 (Chapters 6, 7). **Suction apparatus** is required to clear oropharyngeal secretions. **Laryngoscopes** enable laryngeal visualization (Fig. b). Curved Macintosh and straight Miller blades are most popular. **Endotracheal tubes (ETTs)** should be available in a number of sizes. The usual tube size in adult males is 8–9 mm (internal diameter in mm) and 7–8 mm in adult females. Most ETTs are made of polyvinyl chloride with low-pressure, high-volume cuffs. **Drugs** including anaesthetic, muscle relaxant and vasoactive agents (e.g. atropine, adrenaline) must be readily available. **Monitoring equipment** should include capnography for end-tidal CO_2 measurement.

- **Intubation.** All critically ill patients are assumed to have full stomachs (e.g. emergencies, <8 h or unknown fasting status, trauma) or paralytic ileus (e.g. intestinal obstruction, gastric paresis due to diabetes or opiate analgesia) and are at high risk of aspiration.

Rapid sequence induction (RSI; Fig. b) rapidly secures the airway (i.e. without mask ventilation) and reduces the risk of aspiration in these patients. After preoxygenation, an induction agent (e.g. etomidate, midazolam) is administered, quickly followed by a rapidly acting muscle relaxant (e.g. suxamethonium). Simultaneously an assistant applies anterior pressure to the cricoid cartilage, which closes the oesophagus preventing gastric regurgitation (Sellick manoeuvre). The patient is positioned with the **neck flexed** (i.e. one pillow beneath the occiput) and **head extended** ('sniffing the morning air') to align the glottis, pharynx and oral cavity and achieve the best view on laryngoscopy (Fig. b). Intubation rapidly follows (Fig. b). Cricoid pressure is released only after inflation of the tube cuff. A **modified RSI** using a nondepolarizing muscle relaxant (e.g. atracurium, rocuronium) is recommended in situations where suxamethonium is contraindicated (e.g. renal failure, neuromuscular disorders and >6 h after trauma or burns).

Normal intubation differs from RSI in that the patient is usually stable (i.e. haemodynamically), fasted for >6 h, does not require cricoid pressure, and mask ventilation is established before giving the muscle relaxant, then continued for 2–3 min to ensure complete paralysis before intubation.

- **Awake intubation** is considered for difficult ETIs. Following upper airways topical anaesthesia (e.g. lidocaine, cocaine), sedation and analgesia are titrated so the patient is not obtunded. The ETT is loaded onto a fibreoptic scope and passed into the trachea.

- **Difficult intubation aids** include **gum elastic bougies/flexible stylets** which aid ETI when the tracheal opening is anterior to the visual axis. **Fibreoptic endoscopy** allows direct visualization of intubation. **Light wands** transilluminate the neck at the laryngeal entrance, aiding 'blind' intubation.

- **Failed intubation drill.** If initial intubation attempts fail (<1: 300), summon help. Consider waking the patient, although this may not be an option in emergencies. If mask ventilation is effective, try alternative approaches to intubation (e.g. fibreoptic endoscopy) but maintain cricoid pressure in RSI. If mask ventilation is inadequate, attempt laryngeal mask (Chapter 7) ventilation. If this is unsuccessful, an emergency cricothyroidotomy may be required (Chapters 11, 29).

- **ETI complications** include hypoxaemia, aspiration, bronchospasm and trauma (e.g. teeth, vocal cords, cervical spine).

- **ETT care.** The distance from the lips to the tip of the ETT should be ~22–24 cm. The tube will move ~4 cm from full neck flexion to extension. The right main bronchus is intubated if the ETT is inserted too far, impairing ventilation of the opposite lung. ETT position is checked on CXR. High cuff inflation pressures (>20 cmH$_2$O), oversized ETTs, head movement and prolonged intubation (>7–14 days) are avoided as these cause pressure-induced ischaemic ulcers, granulation tissue and eventually tracheal stenosis. Avoid long ETTs which increase airways resistance.

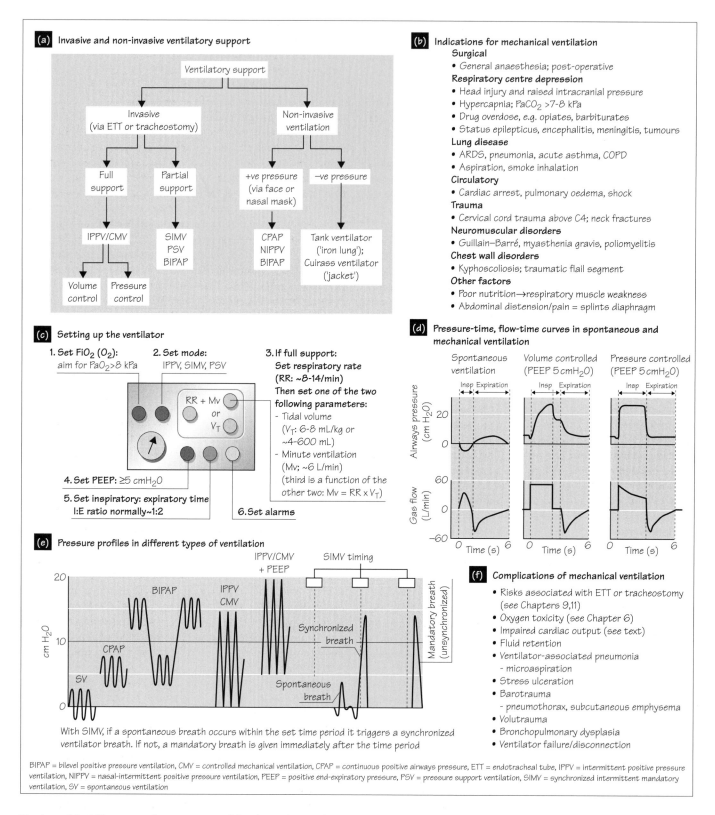

(a) Invasive and non-invasive ventilatory support

(b) Indications for mechanical ventilation
Surgical
- General anaesthesia; post-operative

Respiratory centre depression
- Head injury and raised intracranial pressure
- Hypercapnia; $PaCO_2$ >7-8 kPa
- Drug overdose, e.g. opiates, barbiturates
- Status epilepticus, encephalitis, meningitis, tumours

Lung disease
- ARDS, pneumonia, acute asthma, COPD
- Aspiration, smoke inhalation

Circulatory
- Cardiac arrest, pulmonary oedema, shock

Trauma
- Cervical cord trauma above C4; neck fractures

Neuromuscular disorders
- Guillain–Barré, myasthenia gravis, poliomyelitis

Chest wall disorders
- Kyphoscoliosis; traumatic flail segment

Other factors
- Poor nutrition→respiratory muscle weakness
- Abdominal distension/pain = splints diaphragm

(c) Setting up the ventilator

1. Set FiO_2 (O_2): aim for PaO_2 >8 kPa
2. Set mode: IPPV, SIMV, PSV
3. If full support: Set respiratory rate (RR: ~8-14/min) Then set one of the two following parameters:
   - Tidal volume (V_T: 6-8 mL/kg or ~4-600 mL)
   - Minute ventilation (Mv; ~6 L/min) (third is a function of the other two: $Mv = RR \times V_T$)
4. Set PEEP: ≥5 cmH₂O
5. Set inspiratory: expiratory time I:E ratio normally~1:2
6. Set alarms

(d) Pressure-time, flow-time curves in spontaneous and mechanical ventilation

Spontaneous ventilation
Volume controlled (PEEP 5 cmH₂O)
Pressure controlled (PEEP 5 cmH₂O)

Airways pressure (cm H₂O)
Gas flow (L/min)
Time (s)

(e) Pressure profiles in different types of ventilation

SV, CPAP, BIPAP, IPPV CMV, IPPV/CMV + PEEP, SIMV timing, Synchronized breath, Spontaneous breath, Mandatory breath (unsynchronized)

cm H₂O

With SIMV, if a spontaneous breath occurs within the set time period it triggers a synchronized ventilator breath. If not, a mandatory breath is given immediately after the time period

(f) Complications of mechanical ventilation
- Risks associated with ETT or tracheostomy (see Chapters 9,11)
- Oxygen toxicity (see Chapter 6)
- Impaired cardiac output (see text)
- Fluid retention
- Ventilator-associated pneumonia
  - microaspiration
- Stress ulceration
- Barotrauma
  - pneumothorax, subcutaneous emphysema
- Volutrauma
- Bronchopulmonary dysplasia
- Ventilator failure/disconnection

BIPAP = bilevel positive pressure ventilation, CMV = controlled mechanical ventilation, CPAP = continuous positive airways pressure, ETT = endotracheal tube, IPPV = intermittent positive pressure ventilation, NIPPV = nasal-intermittent positive pressure ventilation, PEEP = positive end-expiratory pressure, PSV = pressure support ventilation, SIMV = synchronized intermittent mandatory ventilation, SV = spontaneous ventilation

During critical illness, ventilatory support (Fig. a) may be required to maintain gas exchange and reduce WoB. Mechanical ventilation (MV) is usually delivered through an endotracheal tube or tra-cheostomy and provides complete or partial respiratory support. Non-invasive ventilation (NIV) aids spontaneous ventilation and avoids the need for endotracheal intubation (Chapter 9).

Indications for MV (Fig. b)

Outside the operating theatre, the main indication for MV is respiratory failure. However, its value in the support of other organs, especially during shock or cardiac failure, is increasingly being recognized. Apart from in acute emergencies (e.g. cardiac arrest), the difficult decision is when and whether to ventilate a progressively deteriorating patient. There are no simple guidelines. However, hypoxaemia ($Po_2 < 8\,kPa$ on $F_io_2 > 0.4$), hypercapnia ($Pco_2 > 7.5\,kPa$), respiratory/metabolic acidosis (pH < 7.2) and physical factors (e.g. confusion, exhaustion, poor cough) usually indicate the need for MV. Trends in these variables are often more helpful than absolute values. MV should only be considered when there is a reasonable chance of survival. In terminal illness, support may be limited to NIV, after appropriate discussion with the patient and/or relatives (Chapter 17).

Ventilator set-up (Fig. c)

Typical initial adult intermittent positive pressure ventilation (IPPV) settings would be: tidal volume (V_T) ~6–8 mL/kg; respiratory frequency (f) ~8–14 breaths/min; and minute ventilation ($M_V = V_T \times f$) ~6 L/min. F_io_2 and M_V are adjusted to maintain $P_ao_2 > 8\,kPa$ and $P_aco_2 < 7\,kPa$, respectively, but acceptable values depend on individual disease processes (Chapters 6, 25). Initially PEEP is set at $\geq 5\,cmH_2O$ and the inspiratory : expiratory time (I : E ratio) at ~1 : 2. Disease-specific ventilatory strategies are discussed in individual chapters.

Mode of ventilation (Fig. e)

Mode of ventilation describes whether a breath is: (i) fully or partially supported; (ii) volume or pressure controlled; (iii) mandatory (delivered by the ventilator regardless of patient respiratory effort); or (iv) spontaneously triggered (Figs a and e). The duration of a breath may be fixed (i.e. timed) or variable (i.e. dependent on tidal volume delivery). Modern ventilators with microprocessor controls provide considerable flexibility, allowing a change from mandatory, full support modes to partial support modes that minimize sedation requirements and allow patients to be conscious but comfortable.

- **Full (mandatory) support modes** (e.g. IPPV, controlled mechanical ventilation (CMV)) are uncomfortable and may require sedation as no allowance is made for spontaneous respiration. They are used in severe respiratory disease, in circulatory instability or when respiratory drive is absent. Volume- and pressure-controlled ventilatory (VCV, PCV) modes are available but the pattern of gas flow in PCV achieves optimal gas exchange.

   Volume-controlled IPPV/CMV (Fig. d) is often used postoperatively. Each breath is delivered at a preset volume over a fixed time. Airway pressure varies with lung compliance.

   Pressure-controlled IPPV/CMV (Fig. d) delivers a preset pressure and there is no direct control of tidal volume, which depends on inspiratory time, lung compliance and airways resistance. PCV protects lungs by limiting peak inspiratory pressures (PIPs) and encourages alveolar recruitment.

- **Partial support modes** reinforce spontaneous ventilation and are preferred when possible, to allow a reduction in sedation. Breaths are initiated by the patient and detected by sensitive flow/pressure triggers in the ventilator, which then provides inspiratory support.

   Assist control. The ventilator delivers a breath when triggered by inspiratory effort or independently if the patient does not breathe within a certain time.

   Synchronized intermittent mandatory ventilation (SIMV) delivers a set number of mechanically imposed breaths to achieve a minimum minute ventilation but allows pressure-supported spontaneous breathing. Imposed breaths are reduced as the patient becomes ventilator independent during weaning.

   Pressure support. A preset pressure supports every spontaneous breath. The rate is dependent on the patient. Gradual pressure reductions make it a comfortable and effective mode of weaning (Chapter 11).

- **Positive end-expiratory pressure (PEEP)** describes a positive pressure, maintained throughout expiration, that increases functional residual capacity (i.e. alveolar recruitment), prevents alveolar collapse at end-expiration, reduces V/Q mismatch and decreases alveolar oedema by increasing lymphatic drainage. PEEP improves oxygenation and oxygen delivery for any given mode of ventilation, provided that CO is not significantly reduced by the associated increase in intrathoracic pressure (IP).

Physiological responses to MV

1 *Cardiovascular effects* are due to increased IP and alveolar overdistension. Increased IP has two effects on the heart.

   (i) Right ventricular (RV) preload reduction is due to increased right atrial pressure, which reduces venous return and RV cardiac output. However, fluid infusion rapidly restores venous return and CO.

   (ii) Left ventricular (LV) afterload reduction is due to reduced LV transmural pressure, which decreases LV work. In the normal heart, any beneficial effect of LV afterload reduction is offset by reduced venous return. However, in the failing heart, CO is relatively insensitive to preload changes but very sensitive to afterload reduction (Chapter 20). Consequently, MV may increase CO in heart failure, a useful therapeutic effect.

The overall response to raised IP depends on the state of the heart, vasomotor tone and fluid status (e.g. hypovolaemia). MV also increases lung volumes. Overinflated alveoli compress alveolar blood vessels, increasing pulmonary vascular resistance and causing pulmonary hypertension. Subsequent RV distension displaces the septum into the LV cavity, reducing LV filling and CO, an effect known as interventricular dependence.

2 *Respiratory effects.* MV reduces WoB, which increases the proportion of CO going to other potentially ischaemic organs. Re-expansion of collapsed lung segments also improves oxygenation. Unfortunately, supine position, reduced surfactant production and ventilation of poorly perfused lung increases V/Q mismatch.

3 *Fluid retention* is due to antidiuretic hormone secretion.

Complications of MV (Fig. f)

Complications are discussed in relevant chapters. **'Barotrauma'** refers to pressure-induced lung damage (e.g. pneumothorax). High PIP ($>35\,cmH_2O$) due to reduced lung compliance (e.g. ARDS) may cause airways disruption and interstitial gas formation. **'Volutrauma'** describes damage to healthy alveoli due to overdistension during recruitment of diseased lung. **'Protective'** ventilation strategies use low tidal volumes (~6 mL/kg) to avoid volutrauma, keep PIP < $35\,cmH_2O$ and maintain alveolar recruitment with PEEP > $5\,cmH_2O$.

11 Respiratory management, weaning and tracheostomy

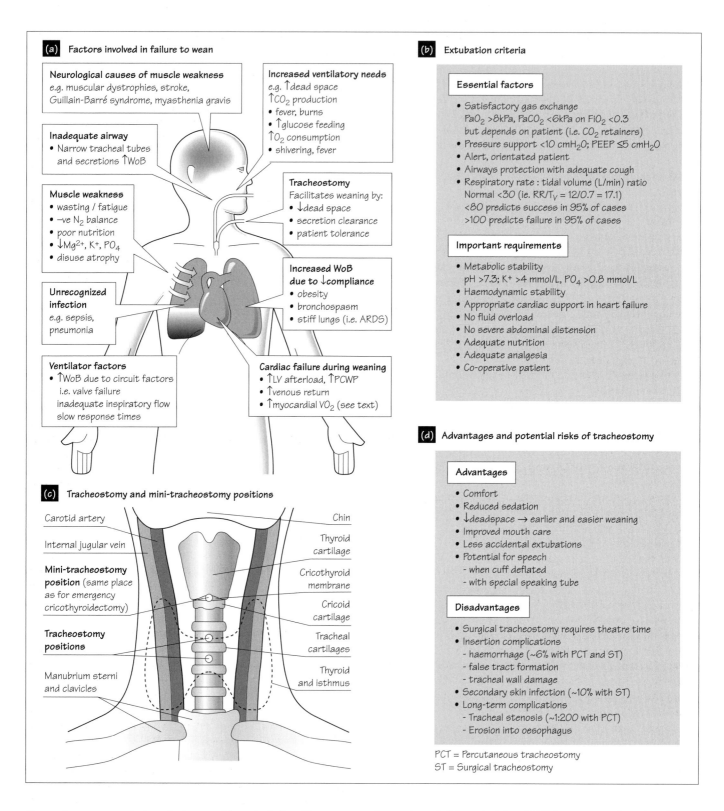

(a) Factors involved in failure to wean

Neurological causes of muscle weakness
e.g. muscular dystrophies, stroke, Guillain-Barré syndrome, myasthenia gravis

Inadequate airway
- Narrow tracheal tubes and secretions ↑WoB

Muscle weakness
- wasting / fatigue
- −ve N_2 balance
- poor nutrition
- ↓Mg^{2+}, K^+, PO_4
- disuse atrophy

Unrecognized infection
e.g. sepsis, pneumonia

Ventilator factors
- ↑WoB due to circuit factors i.e. valve failure inadequate inspiratory flow slow response times

Increased ventilatory needs
e.g. ↑dead space
↑CO_2 production
- fever, burns
- ↑glucose feeding
↑O_2 consumption
- shivering, fever

Tracheostomy
Facilitates weaning by:
- ↓dead space
- secretion clearance
- patient tolerance

Increased WoB due to ↓compliance
- obesity
- bronchospasm
- stiff lungs (i.e. ARDS)

Cardiac failure during weaning
- ↑LV afterload, ↑PCWP
- ↑venous return
- ↑myocardial VO_2 (see text)

(b) Extubation criteria

Essential factors
- Satisfactory gas exchange
  PaO_2 >8kPa, $PaCO_2$ <6kPa on FiO_2 <0.3 but depends on patient (i.e. CO_2 retainers)
- Pressure support <10 cmH₂O; PEEP ≤5 cmH₂O
- Alert, orientated patient
- Airways protection with adequate cough
- Respiratory rate : tidal volume (L/min) ratio Normal <30 (ie. RR/T_V = 12/0.7 = 17.1) <80 predicts success in 95% of cases >100 predicts failure in 95% of cases

Important requirements
- Metabolic stability
  pH >7.3; K^+ >4 mmol/L, PO_4 >0.8 mmol/L
- Haemodynamic stability
- Appropriate cardiac support in heart failure
- No fluid overload
- No severe abdominal distension
- Adequate nutrition
- Adequate analgesia
- Co-operative patient

(c) Tracheostomy and mini-tracheostomy positions

Carotid artery

Internal jugular vein

Mini-tracheostomy position (same place as for emergency cricothyroidectomy)

Tracheostomy positions

Manubrium sterni and clavicles

Chin

Thyroid cartilage

Cricothyroid membrane

Cricoid cartilage

Tracheal cartilages

Thyroid and isthmus

(d) Advantages and potential risks of tracheostomy

Advantages
- Comfort
- Reduced sedation
- ↓deadspace → earlier and easier weaning
- Improved mouth care
- Less accidental extubations
- Potential for speech
  - when cuff deflated
  - with special speaking tube

Disadvantages
- Surgical tracheostomy requires theatre time
- Insertion complications
  - haemorrhage (~6% with PCT and ST)
  - false tract formation
  - tracheal wall damage
- Secondary skin infection (~10% with ST)
- Long-term complications
  - Tracheal stenosis (~1:200 with PCT)
  - Erosion into oesophagus

PCT = Percutaneous tracheostomy
ST = Surgical tracheostomy

General management of respiratory problems includes: (i) oxygen therapy; (ii) secretion clearance; (iii) prompt treatment of infection; (iv) reduction of WoB by improving compliance (e.g. oedema treatment) and decreasing airways resistance (e.g. bronchodilator therapy); and (v) optimizing FRC by encouraging alveolar recruitment (e.g. CPAP) when FRC is low (e.g. pneumonia) and avoiding gas trapping and raised intrathoracic pressure (Chapters 24, 25) when FRC is high (e.g. asthma).

Management of ventilated patients

Important considerations are:
- **Sedation.** Some ventilatory strategies are uncomfortable and sedation (± paralysis) may be required to prevent a patient 'fighting the ventilator'. However, in agitated or restless subjects always exclude other problems (e.g. pneumothorax, pulmonary oedema, pain) before administering sedation.
- **Ventilator dependence.** Control of breathing is abolished in sedated and/or paralysed patients. Ventilator alarms must be set for:
   (i) *Minimum acceptable ventilation* to identify ventilator disconnection/failure.
   (ii) *Maximum acceptable airways pressures* to avoid barotrauma.

Ventilated patients cannot compensate for metabolic derangements (e.g. hyperventilation in acidosis). Therefore, blood gases must be monitored, ventilator settings adjusted and treatment instituted (e.g. bicarbonate infusion) to correct abnormalities.
- **Airways management.** Regular suctioning, physiotherapy and 'turning/positioning' will facilitate secretion clearance and prevent airways obstruction or distal alveolar collapse. Inspired gas is humidified and warmed to minimize viscid secretions. ETT care is essential (Chapter 9). CXR confirms ETT position and monitors ongoing respiratory disease. Bronchoscopy facilitates removal of airways obstructions (e.g. secretions, blood clots), sampling (e.g. microbiology) and investigation (e.g. cause of haemoptysis).
- **Ventilator management** (Chapters 10, 23–29) includes:
   (i) 'Protective' strategies which aim to reduce ventilator-induced damage (e.g. barotrauma) in diseased lungs (e.g. ARDS) that require high distending pressures to achieve normal V_T (i.e. low compliance and FRC due to fibrosis, consolidation, atelectasis). Ventilation with small tidal volumes (~6 mL/kg) and low peak inspiratory pressures (i.e. < 35 cmH_2O) decreases volutrauma and barotrauma, respectively. Increased mean airways pressures (e.g. PEEP) and long I:E ratios (i.e. > 1:1) promote alveolar recruitment and improve oxygenation.
   (ii) 'Asthma' strategies which increase alveolar ventilation and CO_2 clearance by reducing gas trapping when airways resistance or FRC is high (e.g. asthma, COPD). Reduced breathing frequency and low I:E ratios (<1:2) increase expiratory time and hence expiratory volume. Likewise, modest PEEP levels hold open potentially collapsible airways during expiration, increasing expiratory volume. The resulting fall in FRC increases inspiratory volume and minute ventilation.
   (iii) 'Oxygenation' strategies which aim to reduce shunt fraction (Chapter 26). Rarely, **nitric oxide,** an inhaled vasodilator, is used to increase blood flow through ventilated alveolar capillaries, briefly reducing hypoxaemia (~24 h). Likewise, **prone positioning** (i.e. face down) improves oxygenation in >50% of persistently hypoxaemic patients with dependent consolidation by improving V/Q matching and recruiting poorly ventilated basal lung segments. Neither therapy improves survival.

Weaning

Weaning is the process of reducing and then removing respiratory support. It is not usually required in patients who are ventilated for short periods (i.e. postoperative). A simple trial of breathing through the ETT and comparing the ratio of respiratory rate (RR) to tidal volume (V_T; L/min) will determine the likelihood of successful extubation. The normal RR/V_T ratio is <30 (i.e. 12/0.7 = 17.1) and <80 or >100 strongly predicts success or failure, respectively. Weaning is usually required in patients who have been ventilated for long periods with resulting respiratory muscle weakness.

Weaning techniques improve respiratory muscle strength by slowly reducing respiratory support.
1 *Partial support modes* (Chapters 8,10) include:
   (i) Synchronized intermittent mandatory ventilation (SIMV) which allows supported spontaneous breaths between gradually decreasing mandatory (i.e. imposed) breaths.
   (ii) Pressure support (PS) ventilation. PS for patient-triggered breaths is slowly decreased until the patient is doing all the work. A small amount of PS compensates for the work imposed by the ETT and breathing circuit.
   (iii) Bilevel positive pressure ventilation (BIPAP) which delivers two levels of pressure in phase with respiration. The higher pressure provides inspiratory support and augments V_T; the lower pressure is applied during expiration and increases FRC. It can be delivered via an ETT or facemask.
2 *Continuous positive airways pressure* increases FRC, in the same way as PEEP, in a spontaneously breathing patient (Chapter 8). It can be delivered through an ETT or facemask.
3 *Non-invasive ventilation* allows weaning to continue after ETT removal (see Chapter 8).

Potential weaning difficulties are illustrated in Fig. (a). After extubation, cardiac dysfunction and pulmonary oedema may occur due to: (i) increases in LV afterload, pulmonary capillary 'wedge' pressure and venous return (Chapter 10); or (ii) inability to sustain the increased cardiac output and myocardial oxygen consumption required for the additional work of spontaneous breathing. Supporting the heart with diuretics, afterload reduction and inotropes may be necessary (Chapters 5, 20). **Extubation criteria.** Figure (b) lists essential requirements prior to extubation.

Tracheostomy (Fig. c)

Despite the low-pressure, high-volume cuffs used in modern ETTs, prolonged intubation risks damage to the vocal cords and/or tracheal stenosis. Tracheostomy is usually advisable after 7–14 days, or earlier if it is evident that a patient will require prolonged intubation.
- **Advantages and potential risks** are reported in Fig. (d). **Percutaneous tracheostomy,** performed at the bedside, has the advantages of simplicity, low cost, saved theatre time and fewer complications (e.g. infection) when compared with surgical tracheostomy.
- **Tracheostomy tubes** (± cuffs) are available in a variety of sizes and types. Some have inner tubes that facilitate cleaning, reduce obstruction and allow less frequent tube changes (i.e. ~30 days). Others have long flanges for obese necks.
- **Removal** follows a period of cuff deflation and tube capping to ensure respiratory independence. The remaining stoma is covered with an airtight dressing and heals within a few days.
- **Mini-tracheostomy.** A small tube (~5 mm) is inserted through the cricothyroid membrane (Fig. c), through which a suction catheter can be passed. Although of limited value in ICU, they are useful for short-term secretion clearance when cough or conscious level is temporarily impaired in high dependency areas.

(a) Calculating arterial oxygen partial pressure (PaO₂) from the alveolar gas equation

The simplified alveolar gas equation

$$P_{A}O_2 = FiO_2 (P_b - P_{H_2O}) - (1.25 \times PaCO_2)$$

Breathing air at sea-level where $P_b \sim 101\,kPa$

$$P_{A}O_2 = 0.21 (101 - 6.2) - (1.25 \times 5.3)$$
$$= 19.9 - 6.63 = \sim 13\text{-}14\,kPa$$

PaO₂ slightly lower than $P_{A}O_2$ because of normal shunt fraction ($\sim 3\%$) $\sim 12.5\text{-}13\,kPa$

$P_{A}O_2$ (and thus PaO₂) breathing air at 4500 m altitude where Pb $\sim 53\,kPa$ will be $\sim 7\text{-}8\,kPa$

$P_{A}O_2$ = alveolar oxygen tension,
FiO_2 = fractional concentration of oxygen in inspired air,
P_b = barometric pressure,
P_{H_2O} = water vapour pressure (6.2 kPa),
PaO₂ = arterial oxygen tension,
PaCO₂ = arterial CO₂ tension

(b) The bicarbonate buffer system and the Henderson-Hasselbach equation

The bicarbonate buffer system

Carbonic anhydrase
$$CO_2 + H_2O \leftrightarrow H_2CO_3 \leftrightarrow HCO_3^- + H^+$$

The Henderson-Hasselbach equation

$$\rightarrow K = [HCO_3^-] \times [H^+] / [H_2CO_3]$$
From the law of mass action
K = dissociation constant

$$\rightarrow K_A = [HCO_3^-] \times [H^+] / [H_2CO_3]$$
At equilibrium $[CO_2] \, \alpha [H_2CO_3]$
K_A = corrected dissociation constant

$$\rightarrow \log K_A = \log [H^+] + \log ([HCO_3^-] / [CO_2])$$
$$\rightarrow -\log [H^+] = -\log K_A + \log ([HCO_3^-] / [CO_2])$$
$$\rightarrow pH = pK_A + \log ([HCO_3^-] / [CO_2])$$
(Henderson-Hasselbach equation)

(c) The relationship between pH, HCO₃⁻ and PCO₂

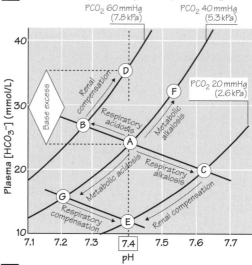

The line BAC is the *buffer line for whole blood*; changes in PCO_2 alter HCO_3^- and pH along this line. Point A represents normal conditions (pH 7.4, HCO_3^- 24 mmol/L, PCO_2 5.3 kPa). An acute rise in PCO_2 (e.g. hypoventilation) decreases the HCO_3^- : PCO_2 ratio and hence pH. This *respiratory acidosis* is represented by a move from A to B. A to C represents a respiratory alkalosis (e.g. hyperventilation). Sustained respiratory acidosis (e.g. chronic respiratory failure) is compensated for by renal HCO_3^- reabsorption and H^+ excretion. The HCO_3^- : PCO_2 ratio is restored and pH returns to normal. This *renal compensation* is described by the arrow B to D. Conversely a respiratory alkalosis may be compensated for by increased renal excretion of HCO_3^- (C to E). Metabolic acidosis (G) may be partially compensated by increased ventilation and a reduction in PCO_2 (G to E). There is little respiratory compensation of metabolic alkalosis(F).

(d) Flenley acid-base nomogram

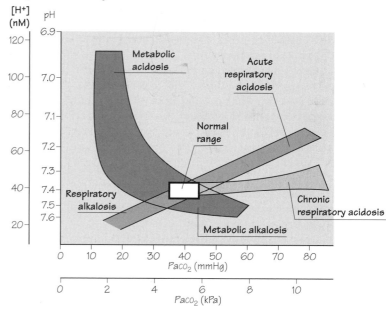

(e) Disorders of acid-base balance

1. Metabolic acidosis

Normal anion gap
• Renal HCO_3^- loss: proximal RTA, tubular damage (e.g. heavy metals)
• Loss of HCO_3^- from the gut: diarrhoea, ileostomy
• Decreased renal H^+ secretion: distal RTA

Increased anion gap; organic acid accumulation
• Lactic acidosis: Type A (sepsis, cardiac arrest, hypotension, methanol), Type B (insulin deficiency, metformin, decreased hepatic metabolism)
• Ketoacidosis: insulin deficiency (e.g. diabetic ketoacidosis), starvation
• Exogenous acids: salicylates

2. Metabolic alkalosis
• H^+ loss: vomiting, renal loss, diuretics, hypokalaemia, low Cl^- states
• HCO_3^- gain: sodium HCO_3^-, lactate, citrate administration

3. Respiratory acidosis
• Airways obstruction, pneumonia, ARDS, pulmonary oedema
• Respiratory muscle weakness: myasthenia, Guillain-Barré, polio
• Trauma: flail segment, lung contusion
• Respiratory depression: head trauma, opiates

4. Respiratory alkalosis
• High levels of anxiety or pain
• Altitude
• Excessive mechanical ventilation
• Respiratory stimulants: salicylate overdose
• Pulmonary embolism, asthma, oedema

HCO_3^- = bicarbonate, H^+ = hydrogen ion, RTA = renal tubular acidosis, Cl^-= chloride ion, ARDS = acute respiratory distress syndrome

Arterial blood gases

Understanding arterial blood gases (ABGs) is essential to the management of critically ill patients. Although certain inferences can be made from ABG data alone, full interpretation requires knowledge of the clinical context, serum electrolyte concentrations and occasionally serum albumin and lactate levels. The blood gas analyser will typically display the following.

1 *Arterial partial pressure of oxygen* ($P_a o_2$), which is measured directly. Its relationship with the fractional inspired oxygen concentration ($F_i o_2$) is described by the alveolar gas equation (Fig. a). When breathing air at sea level (i.e. barometric pressure ~101 kPa), the partial pressure of inspired oxygen ($P_i o_2$) is ~21 kPa. This falls to ~19.9 kPa when fully saturated with water in the upper airways. In the alveolus, O_2 is taken up and replaced with CO_2, which reduces the alveolar oxygen partial pressure ($P_A o_2$) to ~13–14 kPa. The $P_a o_2$ is slightly lower than the $P_A o_2$ due to the normal pulmonary shunt fraction (~3%). Normal $P_a o_2$ is ~13 kPa (~100 mmHg) at the age of 20 years and ~11 kPa at 65 years.

2 *Arterial partial pressure of carbon dioxide* ($P_a co_2$), which is measured directly and is normally ~5.3 kPa (40 mmHg).

3 *pH*, the negative logarithm$_{10}$ of the hydrogen ion concentration ([H^+] = 40 nM).

4 *Standard bicarbonate*, which is calculated from the CO_2 and pH using the Henderson–Hasselbach equation (Fig. b). It is the concentration of bicarbonate [HCO_3^-] in a sample equilibrated to 37°C and $P_a co_2$ 5.3 kPa. It allows assessment of the metabolic component of acid–base balance. Normal values are ~21–27 mmol/L.

5 *Actual bicarbonate*, which reflects the contribution of both respiratory and metabolic components. In venous blood the normal value is 21–28 mmol/L.

6 *Base excess (BE)*, which is a measure of the amount of acid or alkali (in mmol/L) that must be added to a sample, under standard conditions (37°C, $P_a co_2$ 5.3 kPa), to return the pH to 7.4. It quantifies metabolic acid–base status by comparing the 'corrected' HCO_3^- with the 'normal' HCO_3^- (i.e. ~24 mmol/L at pH 7.4). It is calculated automatically from pH and $P_a co_2$ and corrected for haemoglobin. The normal range is +2 mmol/L to –2 mmol/L.

Interpreting arterial blood gases

Having noted the $P_a o_2$ and $F_i o_2$, a simple method for analysing ABG is:

1 *Assess pH.* A pH outside the normal range defines acidaemia (<7.35) or alkalaemia (>7.45).

2 *Assess the respiratory component.* $P_a co_2$ > 6 kPa (45 mmHg) defines respiratory acidosis; $P_a co_2$ < 4.5 kPa (35 mmHg) defines respiratory alkalosis.

3 *Assess the metabolic component.* HCO_3^- > 33 mmol/L defines metabolic alkalosis; HCO_3^- < 23 mmol/L defines metabolic acidosis.

4 *Determine if there is metabolic or respiratory compensation.* See acid–base balance below.

5 *Consider the anion gap (AG).* This is the difference between the sum of serum sodium and potassium ion concentrations and the sum of serum chloride and bicarbonate ion concentrations: [(Na^+) + (K^+)] – [(Cl^-) + (HCO_3^-)]. The normal AG (~10–18 mmol/L) is a reflection of the kidney-excreted mineral acids (e.g. phosphates). An increased AG indicates an accumulation of organic acids including ketoacids, lactic acid and exogenous acids (e.g. salicylates).

Acid–base balance

Maintenance of a stable hydrogen ion concentration (45–35 nM) or pH between 7.35 and 7.45 is essential for intracellular enzyme function. Normally acids are generated by the hydration of CO_2 ('respiratory acids') or other processes of metabolism ('metabolic' acids; typically phosphoric, sulphuric and lactic). In disease states, [H^+] can rise due to lactate production (e.g. ischaemia), ketoacid generation (e.g. diabetes), alcohol ingestion (e.g. methanol) or failure of normal excretion (e.g. renal, respiratory or liver failure). Loss of H^+ (e.g. vomiting) or HCO_3^- (e.g. diarrhoea) also affects acid–base balance. **Causes** are listed in Fig. (e).

Control of acid–base balance

The body prevents pH changes by regulating two pathways for eliminating acid: respiratory and renal. However, ~100 times more acid equivalents are expired each day in the form of CO_2/carbonic acid than are excreted as fixed acids by the kidneys. **Buffers** bind or release H^+ according to the pH; this limits the change in pH that occurs when acid is added. The relationship between the amount of acid added to a buffer-containing solution and the change in pH is known as the **buffer line**. Buffers are most effective when pH is close to their pK_A (log of the dissociation constant K_A; Fig. b). The most important blood buffer systems are:

1 *Bicarbonate* (HCO_3^-; Fig. b). CO_2 combines with water to form carbonic acid (H_2CO_3) which dissociates to HCO_3^- and H^+. The relationship between pH, Pco_2 and [HCO_3^-] is described by the Henderson–Hasselbalch equation. In normal blood, [HCO_3^-] is 24 mmol/L, Pco_2 5.3 kPa and pH calculates to 7.4. If the ratio [HCO_3^-] : Pco_2 remains at 20, pH will remain at 7.4. Although the pK_A of the bicarbonate system (6.1) is further away from the blood pH (7.4) than would seem ideal for a buffer, the fact that Pco_2 and HCO_3^- can be independently controlled by ventilation and the kidneys, respectively, means that in practice it makes an effective buffer system.

2 *Haemoglobin (Hb)*, particularly when deoxygenated. It significantly improves buffering capacity in whole blood compared with plasma. All other blood proteins have <20% of the buffering capacity of Hb.

The relationship between pH, HCO_3^- and Pco_2

This is illustrated using Davenport diagrams (Fig. c). Acute CO_2 changes cause **respiratory acidosis or alkalosis**. When CO_2 changes persist (e.g. type 2 respiratory failure), pH is slowly corrected by renal compensation (i.e. increased/decreased [HCO_3^-]). The terms **metabolic acidosis and alkalosis** are used to describe alterations in acid–base status due to changes in HCO_3^- rather than CO_2 — as a result, for example, of renal disease or increased H^+ production (e.g. diabetic ketoacidosis). A metabolic acidosis may be partially compensated by increased ventilation. However, there is little respiratory compensation for a metabolic alkalosis which may require unsustainable falls in ventilation. **Mixed metabolic and respiratory** acid–base disorders may occur. For example, respiratory acidosis due to respiratory failure (i.e. increased Pco_2) may be combined with a metabolic acidosis due to the associated hypoxia. The **Flenley nomogram** is a useful diagnostic aid as only one type of disturbance is likely if pH and Pco_2 fall within a specific band (Fig. d).

13 Sedation, analgesia and paralysis

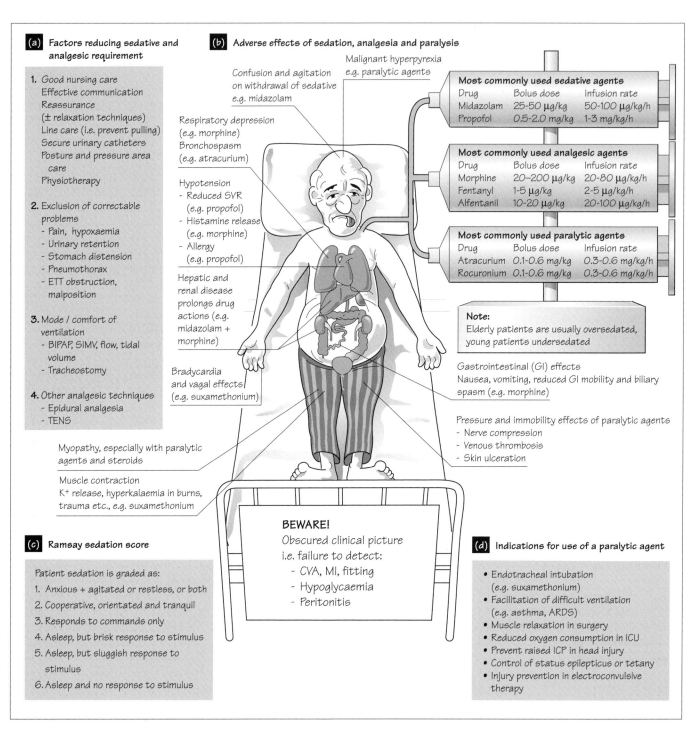

(a) Factors reducing sedative and analgesic requirement

1. Good nursing care
   Effective communication
   Reassurance
   (± relaxation techniques)
   Line care (i.e. prevent pulling)
   Secure urinary catheters
   Posture and pressure area
       care
   Physiotherapy

2. Exclusion of correctable
   problems
   - Pain, hypoxaemia
   - Urinary retention
   - Stomach distension
   - Pneumothorax
   - ETT obstruction,
     malposition

3. Mode / comfort of
   ventilation
   - BIPAP, SIMV, flow, tidal
     volume
   - Tracheostomy

4. Other analgesic techniques
   - Epidural analgesia
   - TENS

(b) Adverse effects of sedation, analgesia and paralysis

Confusion and agitation on withdrawal of sedative e.g. midazolam

Malignant hyperpyrexia e.g. paralytic agents

Respiratory depression (e.g. morphine)
Bronchospasm (e.g. atracurium)

Hypotension
- Reduced SVR
  (e.g. propofol)
- Histamine release
  (e.g. morphine)
- Allergy
  (e.g. propofol)

Hepatic and renal disease prolongs drug actions (e.g. midazolam + morphine)

Bradycardia and vagal effects (e.g. suxamethonium)

Myopathy, especially with paralytic agents and steroids

Muscle contraction
K⁺ release, hyperkalaemia in burns, trauma etc., e.g. suxamethonium

Gastrointestinal (GI) effects
Nausea, vomiting, reduced GI mobility and biliary spasm (e.g. morphine)

Pressure and immobility effects of paralytic agents
- Nerve compression
- Venous thrombosis
- Skin ulceration

Most commonly used sedative agents

Drug	Bolus dose	Infusion rate
Midazolam	25-50 µg/kg	50-100 µg/kg/h
Propofol	0.5-2.0 mg/kg	1-3 mg/kg/h

Most commonly used analgesic agents

Drug	Bolus dose	Infusion rate
Morphine	20-200 µg/kg	20-80 µg/kg/h
Fentanyl	1-5 µg/kg	2-5 µg/kg/h
Alfentanil	10-20 µg/kg	20-100 µg/kg/h

Most commonly used paralytic agents

Drug	Bolus dose	Infusion rate
Atracurium	0.1-0.6 mg/kg	0.3-0.6 mg/kg/h
Rocuronium	0.1-0.6 mg/kg	0.3-0.6 mg/kg/h

Note:
Elderly patients are usually oversedated, young patients undersedated

BEWARE!
Obscured clinical picture
i.e. failure to detect:
- CVA, MI, fitting
- Hypoglycaemia
- Peritonitis

(c) Ramsay sedation score

Patient sedation is graded as:
1. Anxious + agitated or restless, or both
2. Cooperative, orientated and tranquil
3. Responds to commands only
4. Asleep, but brisk response to stimulus
5. Asleep, but sluggish response to stimulus
6. Asleep and no response to stimulus

(d) Indications for use of a paralytic agent

- Endotracheal intubation
  (e.g. suxamethonium)
- Facilitation of difficult ventilation
  (e.g. asthma, ARDS)
- Muscle relaxation in surgery
- Reduced oxygen consumption in ICU
- Prevent raised ICP in head injury
- Control of status epilepticus or tetany
- Injury prevention in electroconvulsive
  therapy

Effective relief of pain and anxiety is essential in critically ill patients. Sedation requirements vary according to the patient's psychology, pathology, therapy, surgery and need for invasive monitoring or mechanical ventilation. Good nursing care, correction of reversible problems, comfortable modes of ventilation, tracheostomy and epidural analgesia reduce drug doses and side-effects (Fig. a). Therapeutic aims are that:

1 *Non-paralysed patients* should be comfortable but able to communicate and cooperate. Heavy sedation is occasionally required for unpleasant ventilatory modes (e.g. inverse I : E ratio), seizure therapy and intracranial pressure reduction. The level of sedation must be assessed regularly, particularly when sedatives are given by infusion. Of the many sedation scoring systems, Ramsay's Scale (Fig. c) is the most frequently used. Levels 2–5 are appropriate for most patients. The adverse effects of excessive sedation are illustrated in Fig. (b). Conversely, unrelieved pain and/or anxiety causes hypertension, tachycardia, atelectasis, immobility, venous thromboembolism and reduced immune function.

2 *Paralysed patients* must always be sedated to unconsciousness. Distress in 'awake' paralysed patients can only be recognized as hypertension, tachycardia, sweating and lacrimation. Limited EEG helps confirm adequate sedation. A peripheral nerve stimulator provides the best index of level of paralysis. The aim is to prevent complete obliteration of 'train of four' electrical stimuli. Paralytic agents should only be used occasionally (Table d) and with great care as unrecognized extubation is fatal.

No drug fulfils the properties of an ideal sedative (i.e. anxiolysis, analgesia, amnesia, predictability, titratability, minimal side-effects and rapid elimination). A multidrug approach using analgesics, sedative-anxiolytic and paralysing agents is required. Choice depends on patient requirements, drug properties and side-effects. Most are administered as bolus or continuous intravenous infusions and titrated to the required effect.

Analgesics
Opioids
Morphine provides potent, rapid-onset analgesia and anxiolysis with minimal cardiovascular instability. High doses (± benzodiazepines) are required to produce unconsciousness. Reduced respiratory drive helps intubated patients synchronize with ventilators but excessive doses cause apnoea. Associated nausea, vomiting and decreased gastrointestinal motility hamper enteral nutrition. Occasional biliary spasm and histamine release occur. Hepatic metabolism precedes renal excretion, and opiates (and metabolites) accumulate in liver and renal failure.

Fentanyl, a synthetic opioid, has a short duration of action after single doses. Accumulation in lipophilic tissue occurs with chronic use. This redistribution, with subsequent slow release from fat stores, rather than clearance failure may result in prolonged action. **Alfentanil** is shorter acting and clearance without redistribution makes accumulation less likely. **Remifentanil**, a new, short-acting agent, requires further assessment. **Naloxone** is an effective but short-acting opioid antagonist.

Paracetamol and non-steroidal anti-inflammatory drugs (NSAID)
Paracetamol is a mild analgesic and antipyretic. Regular administration has an opioid-sparing effect. NSAID inhibit cyclooxygenases (COX) and are effective analgesics alone or synergistically with narcotics. Renal toxicity and GI bleeding limit NSAID use. Unfortunately, paracetamol and most NSAID (with the exception of a few COX-2 inhibitors) cannot be given intravenously.

Sedative-anxiolytics
Benzodiazepines
Benzodiazepines provide excellent sedation, anxiolysis and amnesia with minimal cardiorespiratory effects. They have no analgesic properties but may decrease analgesic requirements by relieving anxiety. Anticonvulsant and muscle relaxing properties are important.

Midazolam is highly lipid soluble, allowing a rapid onset of action (i.e. blood–brain barrier penetration), but accumulation in fat prolongs drug withdrawal. As consciousness returns, the patient may appear confused and disinhibited because dissociative effects linger. Haloperidol controls this situation whereas further mida-

zolam therapy prolongs the agitation. Metabolism and excretion occur in the liver and hepatic disease prolongs drug action. Conversely, patients with liver enzyme induction (alcoholics, epileptics) may require large doses to achieve therapeutic effects. **Lorazepam** is the exception, as it has no hepatic metabolism or active metabolites. **Flumazenil** is a short-acting benzodiazepine antagonist but may precipitate withdrawal (e.g. fitting).

Propofol
Propofol is an easily titrated sedative, with no analgesic properties, short duration of action and rapid drug withdrawal (i.e. reversibility). Hypotension due to reduced systemic vascular resistance occurs in 30% of patients, limiting use in haemodynamic instability. The drug vehicle (i.e. egg and soyabean emulsion) can cause allergic reactions and supports bacterial growth that may cause nosocomial infection. Infusions must be prepared under sterile conditions and changed at short intervals. Metabolism is neither hepatic or renal.

Other sedative-anxiolytics
A combination of haloperidol and benzodiazepine is usually better than either agent alone in severely agitated patients. Barbiturates and phenothiazines have few advantages over other sedatives and cause side-effects (e.g. dystonic reactions).

Neuromuscular paralytic agents
Depolarizing neuromuscular blockers
Depolarizing neuromuscular blockers resemble acetylcholine (ACH) and cause neuromuscular junction (NMJ) depolarization but are not metabolized by acetylcholinesterases. Depolarization continues until the blocker diffuses out of the NMJ where it is degraded by plasma cholinesterase. **Suxamethonium/succinylcholine** has a rapid onset (seconds) and short duration of action (<10 min). It is ideal for intubation. Depolarization causes muscle contraction and K^+ release. This limits ICU use, particularly in renal failure, because hyperkalaemia can occur (e.g. rhabdomyolysis, burns, trauma). Vagal stimulation and bradycardia prevent use of continuous infusions.

Non-depolarizing neuromuscular blockers
Non-depolarizing neuromuscular blockers passively occupy ACH binding sites, prevent ACH action and block depolarization. They have a slow onset (2–3 min) but longer duration of action (e.g. 20–60 min). **Atracurium** and **rocuronium** are non-cumulative and are often used in ICU. Prolonged therapeutic paralysis, particularly with steroid therapy, may result in severe myopathy. Vagal blockade occurs (e.g. pancuronium) and histamine release can precipitate life-threatening bronchospasm (e.g. atracurium).

Many factors potentiate (e.g. acidosis, hyponatraemia, gentamicin, myasthenia gravis) and inhibit (e.g. oedema, prolonged use, phenytoin) neuromuscular blockade. **Pseudocholinesterase deficiency** occurs in 1 in 2500 people and extends the duration of paralysis to 6–8 h. **Complications of paralysis** are illustrated in Fig. (b). **Malignant hyperthermia** is a genetic disorder occasionally precipitated by neuromuscular blockers. Muscular rigidity, fever, raised metabolic rate and metabolic acidosis occur. Lethal cardiac ischaemia and arrhythmias develop if untreated. Intravenous dantrolene is the treatment of choice.

14 Enteral and parenteral nutrition

(a) Nutritional requirements

Normal nutritional requirements

Energy (calorie) requirement

Determined from:
(a) predictive formula (e.g. Harris-Benedict) based on height, weight + gender;
(b) bedside calorimetry: measures O_2 consumption + CO_2 production;
(c) lean body weight

Normally ~30 kcal/kg/day, increasing to >60 kcal/kg/day in severe stress (e.g. burns). Non-protein sources supply ~80% of calories (e.g. carbohydrate 30-70%, fat 15-30%)

Protein requirement

Determined from 24-h urinary nitrogen loss

Nitrogen intake should be ~0.2 g/kg/day, given as protein ~1.5 g/kg/day

Vitamin and trace elements

Serve key physiological and metabolic roles

Nutritional requirements in disease states

Starvation
Electrolyte depletion (PO_4^-, K^+, Mg^{2+}) and glucose intolerance result in impaired cardiac contractility and respiratory muscle function. Electrolyte and glucose imbalance must be corrected. Re-feeding syndrome occurs after prolonged starvation

Renal failure (RF)
High energy feed is used (i.e. 2 kcal/mL) to reduce volume. In TPN essential amino acids (AA) may stimulate protein synthesis and reduce urea by recycling nitrogen into non-essential AA. Low Na^+, low K^+ and supplemental vitamins may be required

COPD
Malnutrition is common. Ventilation in respiratory failure has a high energy expenditure. Overfeeding with carbohydrate causes high CO_2 production. Feeds should contain less carbohydrate and more fat. Fat oxidation produces 30% less CO_2

Hepatic failure
Impaired fat metabolism and carbohydrate intolerance are common. Use of branched chain (instead of aromatic) AA may improve mental status in hepatic encephalopathy. TPN must contain less sodium and volume due to aldosterone-induced water retention

(b) Complications of enteral and parenteral nutrition

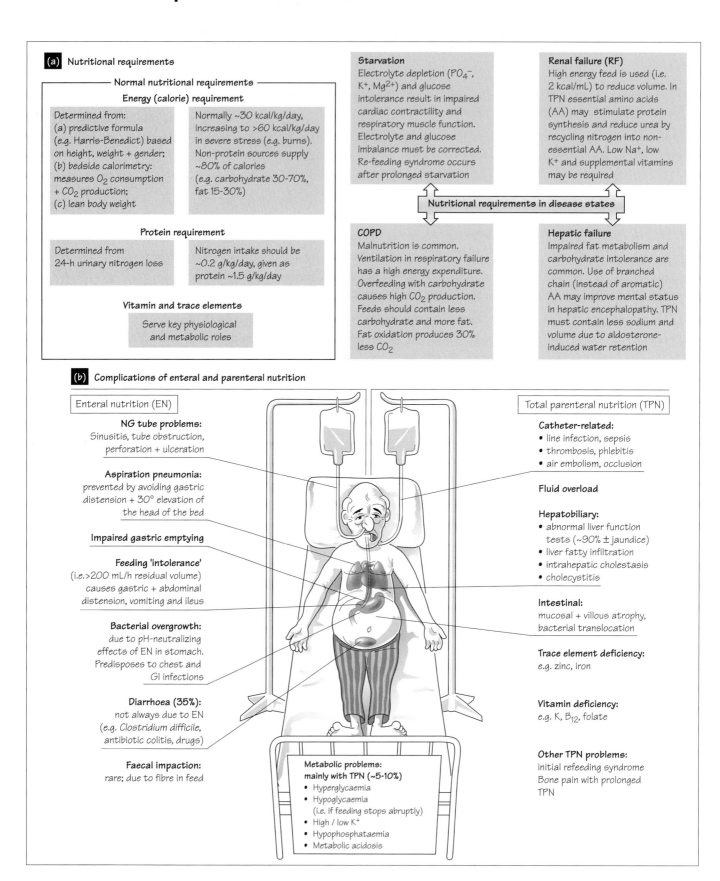

Enteral nutrition (EN)

NG tube problems:
Sinusitis, tube obstruction, perforation + ulceration

Aspiration pneumonia:
prevented by avoiding gastric distension + 30° elevation of the head of the bed

Impaired gastric emptying

Feeding 'intolerance'
(i.e.>200 mL/h residual volume) causes gastric + abdominal distension, vomiting and ileus

Bacterial overgrowth:
due to pH-neutralizing effects of EN in stomach. Predisposes to chest and GI infections

Diarrhoea (35%):
not always due to EN (e.g. *Clostridium difficile*, antibiotic colitis, drugs)

Faecal impaction:
rare; due to fibre in feed

Metabolic problems:
mainly with TPN (~5-10%)
- Hyperglycaemia
- Hypoglycaemia (i.e. if feeding stops abruptly)
- High / low K^+
- Hypophosphataemia
- Metabolic acidosis

Total parenteral nutrition (TPN)

Catheter-related:
- line infection, sepsis
- thrombosis, phlebitis
- air embolism, occlusion

Fluid overload

Hepatobiliary:
- abnormal liver function tests (~90% ± jaundice)
- liver fatty infiltration
- intrahepatic cholestasis
- cholecystitis

Intestinal:
mucosal + villous atrophy, bacterial translocation

Trace element deficiency:
e.g. zinc, iron

Vitamin deficiency:
e.g. K, B_{12}, folate

Other TPN problems:
initial refeeding syndrome Bone pain with prolonged TPN

Assessment of nutrition is essential. Malnutrition impairs immune function, reduces plasma protein and oncotic pressure, delays wound healing and impairs respiratory muscle strength. In critical illness, nutritional support reduces protein catabolism and improves markers of nutritional status (e.g. lymphocyte counts, plasma proteins). However, no specific nutritional regime substantially improves outcome, and complications can outweigh benefits.

Early nutritional support is recommended for pre-existing malnutrition, hypermetabolic states and protracted illness, but is unnecessary in well-nourished, short-stay patients. Figure (a) illustrates typical **nutritional requirements** and adjustments required for COPD, renal and hepatic failure.

Enteral nutrition

Enteral nutrition is always preferred. It increases splanchnic perfusion, preserves mucosal integrity, prevents stress ulceration and bacterial translocation (± sepsis), enhances immunity, supplies complex nutrients (e.g. fibre, medium-chain fatty acids) and stimulates insulin secretion which reduces hyperglycaemia associated with nutritional support. Release of gastrin and other gut hormones promotes pancreatic secretion and gallbladder emptying.

Feeding formulas

Standard commercial feeds provide 1–1.5 kcal/mL (~45% carbohydrate, ~25% lipid) and most electrolyte, vitamin and trace element requirements. They are isotonic, polymeric (i.e. complex protein, fat and carbohydrate molecules) and gluten/lactose free, which reduces the potential for diarrhoea. Elemental diets (i.e. amino acids, oligosaccharides) require minimal digestion (e.g. chronic pancreatitis).

Administration is usually by continuous infusion through a nasogastric tube. Feeding rest periods prevent stomach bacterial overgrowth by allowing restoration of normal gastric pH (<7.1) and reduce the risk of nosocomial pneumonia. Enteral nutrition can be achieved in most patients despite abdominal distension, absence of bowel sounds, diarrhoea or gastric residual volumes >200 mL. Contraindications to enteral nutrition include intestinal obstruction, ischaemia and anatomical disruption. Figure (b) illustrates complications of enteral nutrition. Impaired gastric emptying is managed with prokinetic agents or by bypassing the stomach and feeding directly into the small bowel (e.g. nasojejunal or surgical jejunostomy tubes).

Prokinetic agents promote gastric emptying by activating motilin receptors (e.g. erythromycin) or antagonizing dopamine (e.g. metoclopramide).

Total parenteral nutrition

'Total' parenteral nutrition is required if enteral nutrition is contraindicated or repeated attempts to establish enteral nutrition fail (e.g. ileus, intractable diarrhoea). Benefit from total parenteral nutrition has not been convincingly established. The main energy source in total parenteral nutrition is fat emulsion which causes less metabolic derangement than glucose. Nitrogen is supplied as amino acids. Total parenteral nutrition is nutritionally incomplete, hyperosmolar and irritant.

Most solutions are prepared aseptically in hospital pharmacies, usually as a single bag which is infused into a central vein over 24 h. When total parenteral nutrition is given into a peripheral vein, large volumes with low glucose concentrations are required to reduce osmolality-induced phlebitis. Nevertheless, new line sites may still be required at 2–3-day intervals.

Complications of total parenteral nutrition are listed in Fig. (b). Catheter-related sepsis is reduced using antimicrobial-coated lines, a dedicated lumen and strict aseptic handling. Subcutaneous tunnelling is not of benefit. Insulin may be added to total parenteral nutrition to ensure normoglycaemia. Severe liver dysfunction is reduced by decreasing total parenteral nutrition glucose content.

Immunonutrition

Immunonutrition may improve outcome in critical illness.
- **Glutamine**, an amino acid and primary energy source for enterocytes, preserves intestinal integrity.
- **Arginine** stimulates immune (e.g. T-cell) function and nitrogen balance.
- **Omega-3-polyunsaturated fatty acids**, from fish oils, are anti-inflammatory agents and immune modulators.

15 Hypothermia and hyperthermia

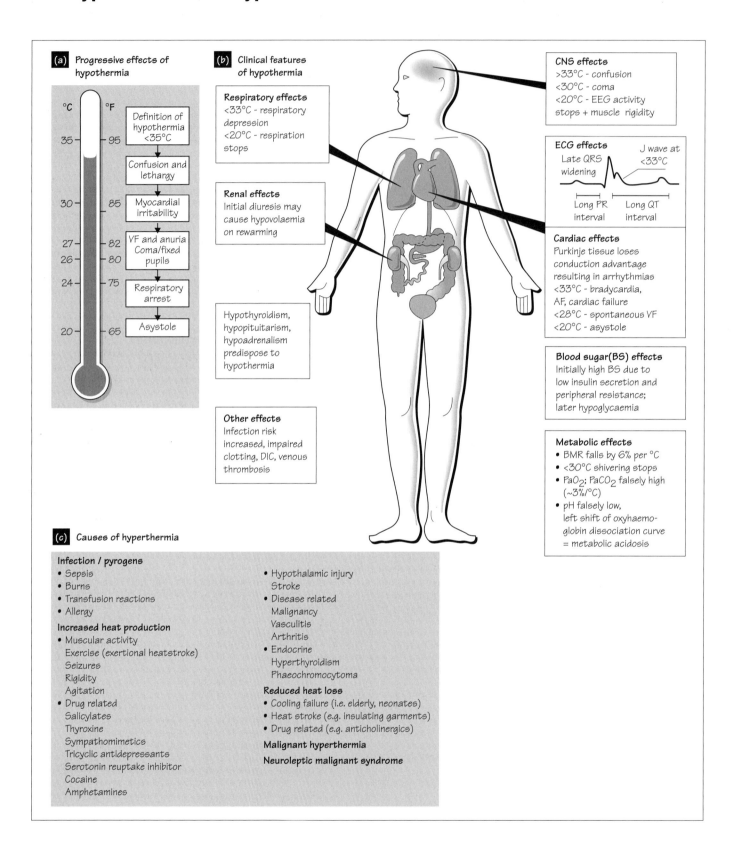

(a) Progressive effects of hypothermia

°C	°F	
35	95	Definition of hypothermia <35°C
		↓
		Confusion and lethargy
30	85	Myocardial irritability
27	82	VF and anuria Coma/fixed pupils
26	80	
24	75	Respiratory arrest
20	65	Asystole

(b) Clinical features of hypothermia

Respiratory effects
<33°C - respiratory depression
<20°C - respiration stops

Renal effects
Initial diuresis may cause hypovolaemia on rewarming

Hypothyroidism, hypopituitarism, hypoadrenalism predispose to hypothermia

Other effects
Infection risk increased, impaired clotting, DIC, venous thrombosis

CNS effects
>33°C - confusion
<30°C - coma
<20°C - EEG activity stops + muscle rigidity

ECG effects
Late QRS widening
J wave at <33°C
Long PR interval
Long QT interval

Cardiac effects
Purkinje tissue loses conduction advantage resulting in arrhythmias
<33°C - bradycardia, AF, cardiac failure
<28°C - spontaneous VF
<20°C - asystole

Blood sugar(BS) effects
Initially high BS due to low insulin secretion and peripheral resistance; later hypoglycaemia

Metabolic effects
- BMR falls by 6% per °C
- <30°C shivering stops
- PaO_2; $PaCO_2$ falsely high (~3%/°C)
- pH falsely low, left shift of oxyhaemo-globin dissociation curve = metabolic acidosis

(c) Causes of hyperthermia

Infection / pyrogens
- Sepsis
- Burns
- Transfusion reactions
- Allergy

Increased heat production
- Muscular activity
  Exercise (exertional heatstroke)
  Seizures
  Rigidity
  Agitation
- Drug related
  Salicylates
  Thyroxine
  Sympathomimetics
  Tricyclic antidepressants
  Serotonin reuptake inhibitor
  Cocaine
  Amphetamines

- Hypothalamic injury
  Stroke
- Disease related
  Malignancy
  Vasculitis
  Arthritis
- Endocrine
  Hyperthyroidism
  Phaeochromocytoma

Reduced heat loss
- Cooling failure (i.e. elderly, neonates)
- Heat stroke (e.g. insulating garments)
- Drug related (e.g. anticholinergics)

Malignant hyperthermia

Neuroleptic malignant syndrome

Hypothermia

Hypothermia is defined as a core temperature <35°C. It affects ~3% of elderly patients admitted to hospital. Mortality varies (i.e. hypothermia alone <10%; with an underlying cause >60%).

Causes

Accidental hypothermia is usually multifactorial, involving exposure to low environmental or water immersion temperatures (e.g. drowning), alcohol intoxication, a primary neurological insult (e.g. cerebrovascular accident), thermoregulatory compromise (e.g. spinal cord injury), predisposing factors (e.g. hypothyroidism, hypopituitarism) and drugs that alter cold perception, cause vasodilation or inhibit heat generation (e.g. barbiturates). Induced hypothermia during cardiac or neurosurgery provides cerebral protection.

Clinical features

Progressive physiological dysfunction affects most organ systems as temperature falls (Fig. a). Cardiorespiratory and neurological failure occur at <30°C. Figure (b) illustrates the clinical features.

General management

General management includes oxygen therapy, prevention of further heat loss and treatment of underlying causes. Rough handling and tracheal intubation may precipitate life-threatening arrhythmias which can be resistant to therapy. Although cardiac resuscitation is performed as normal, cardioversion is often ineffective below 30°C and has to await rewarming.

Rewarming

Caution is required when reversing physiologically well-tolerated hypothermia. Above 33°C, **passive, external rewarming** (i.e. a warm environment and insulating covers) is usually adequate. The use of **active, external rewarming** (i.e. hot water immersion, warming blankets) is controversial as recent reports suggest that peripheral vasodilation aggravates organ hypoperfusion and increases mortality. **Internal rewarming** is indicated in severe hypothermia (<33°C) with poor physiological tolerance or cardiac arrest. Techniques include warm intravenous fluids or inhaled gas, warm gastric, bladder or pleural lavages and haemodialysis or peritoneal lavage (which also remove toxins or drugs). Cardiopulmonary bypass is rarely necessary but can rapidly rewarm during cardiac arrests.

Hyperthermia

Hyperthermia is defined as a core temperature >37.5°C (99°F) and, if severe (>40°C), is potentially lethal. It is associated with increased metabolic rate, CO_2 production and metabolic acidosis. Sweating and vasodilation cause relative hypovolaemia. Epilepsy, neurological impairment, acute renal failure, rhabdomyolysis and myocardial ischaemia may follow.

Causes

Causes are listed in Fig. (c).

Heat stroke affects the elderly and patients with thermoregulatory disorders (e.g. hypothalamic stroke) or inability to dissipate heat (e.g. heart failure, skin disease) during hot weather. Extreme exercise, confined garments and hot environments (e.g. fire fighters) are potential causes.

Drug-induced hyperthermia may be due to serotonin receptor stimulation by amphetamine derivatives (e.g. methylene dioxymethamphetamine (MDMA; 'ecstasy')), serotonin reuptake inhibitors (e.g. fluoxetine, imipramine) or serotonin agonists (e.g. lithium).

Malignant hyperthermia (MH), a rare autosomal dominant trait, causes excessive muscle heat production due to altered calcium kinetics. Muscle rigidity, sudden hyperpyrexia (41–45°C), tachycardia, metabolic acidosis and hypercapnia occur during or shortly after anaesthetic drug exposure. Halothane and suxamethonium/succinylcholine precipitate 80% of cases.

Neuroleptic malignant syndrome (NMS) is an idiosyncratic reaction to neuroleptic drug therapy (e.g. phenothiazines), probably due to hypothalamic antidopaminergic effects. Catatonia, extrapyramidal and autonomic effects are common.

Management

Management includes stopping precipitating drugs, fluid replacement, correction of hyperkalaemia, renal replacement therapy and seizure prophylaxis.

Cooling. Exposure, skin wetting and fans are most effective. Ice packs (e.g. axilla, neck, groin) may be useful. Cold water immersion hampers heat loss due to cutaneous vasoconstriction. Additional measures include cold intravenous fluids, iced gastric or peritoneal lavage, haemofiltration and cardiopulmonary bypass.

Drug therapy

Paracetamol (±NSAID) is often ineffective.

Dantrolene, a muscle relaxant that uncouples the excitation–contraction mechanism, is the definitive treatment for MH, NMS and MDMA. Bromocriptine, anticholinergics and muscle relaxants may also be required.

Mannitol reduces myoglobin-induced renal damage.

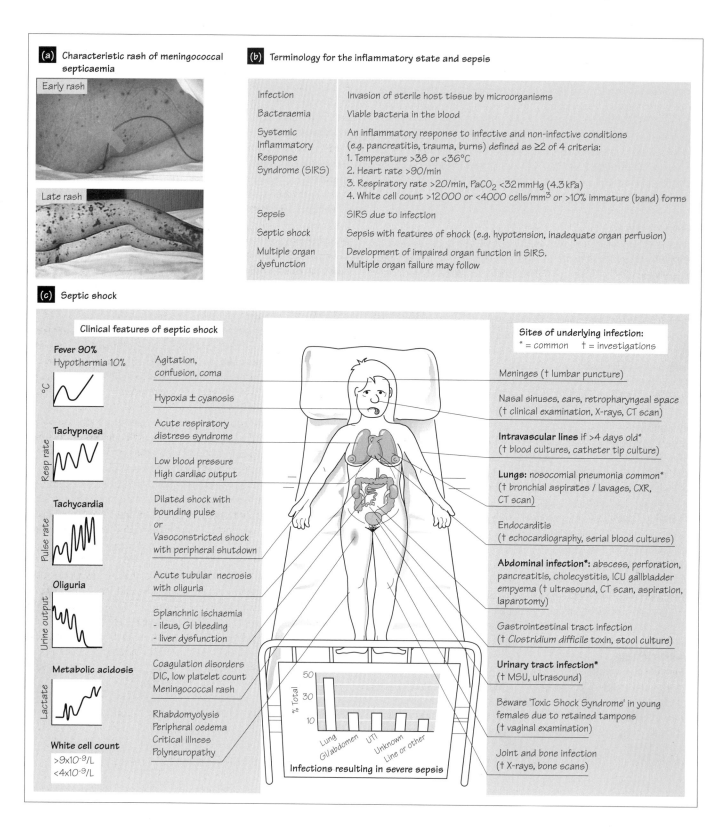

(a) Characteristic rash of meningococcal septicaemia

Early rash

Late rash

(b) Terminology for the inflammatory state and sepsis

Infection	Invasion of sterile host tissue by microorganisms
Bacteraemia	Viable bacteria in the blood
Systemic Inflammatory Response Syndrome (SIRS)	An inflammatory response to infective and non-infective conditions (e.g. pancreatitis, trauma, burns) defined as ≥2 of 4 criteria: 1. Temperature >38 or <36°C 2. Heart rate >90/min 3. Respiratory rate >20/min, $PaCO_2$ <32 mmHg (4.3 kPa) 4. White cell count >12 000 or <4000 cells/mm³ or >10% immature (band) forms
Sepsis	SIRS due to infection
Septic shock	Sepsis with features of shock (e.g. hypotension, inadequate organ perfusion)
Multiple organ dysfunction	Development of impaired organ function in SIRS. Multiple organ failure may follow

(c) Septic shock

Clinical features of septic shock

Fever 90%
Hypothermia 10%

Tachypnoea

Tachycardia

Oliguria

Metabolic acidosis

White cell count
>9x10⁻⁹/L
<4x10⁻⁹/L

Agitation, confusion, coma

Hypoxia ± cyanosis

Acute respiratory distress syndrome

Low blood pressure
High cardiac output

Dilated shock with bounding pulse
or
Vasoconstricted shock with peripheral shutdown

Acute tubular necrosis with oliguria

Splanchnic ischaemia
- ileus, GI bleeding
- liver dysfunction

Coagulation disorders
DIC, low platelet count
Meningococcal rash

Rhabdomyolysis
Peripheral oedema
Critical illness
Polyneuropathy

Sites of underlying infection:
* = common   † = investigations

Meninges († lumbar puncture)

Nasal sinuses, ears, retropharyngeal space († clinical examination, X-rays, CT scan)

Intravascular lines if >4 days old*
(† blood cultures, catheter tip culture)

Lungs: nosocomial pneumonia common*
(† bronchial aspirates / lavages, CXR, CT scan)

Endocarditis
(† echocardiography, serial blood cultures)

Abdominal infection*: abscess, perforation, pancreatitis, cholecystitis, ICU gallbladder empyema († ultrasound, CT scan, aspiration, laparotomy)

Gastrointestinal tract infection
(† Clostridium difficile toxin, stool culture)

Urinary tract infection*
(† MSU, ultrasound)

Beware 'Toxic Shock Syndrome' in young females due to retained tampons
(† vaginal examination)

Joint and bone infection
(† X-rays, bone scans)

Infections resulting in severe sepsis
Lung
GI/abdomen
UTI
Unknown
Line or other
% Total
50
30
10

Definitions. The inflammatory response that characterizes the 'septic state' is not always due to infection. A potential infective cause is detected in ~60–70% of severe sepsis cases but blood cultures are positive in <25%. Figure (b) presents the current terminology used to describe infection, SIRS, sepsis and septic shock.
Epidemiology. Infection and sepsis cause significant morbidity

and mortality on critical care units; at any one time ~50% of patients are on antibiotics, and infection was acquired after admission in about half. In the USA, ~500000 patients, with an average age of 55 years, develop sepsis each year. It is the leading cause of multiple organ failure, ARDS, acute renal failure and late death following trauma. **Prognosis** deteriorates with age, lactic acidosis, low white cell count, cytokine elevation, reduced SVR and number of organ failures. **Mortality** is ~40–60% in septic shock.

Pathophysiology

Septic shock is a major cause of **multiorgan dysfunction**. The **host's immune response** is stimulated by invasive microorganisms or bacterial endotoxins (Chapter 4). Initial cytokine release (e.g. tumour necrosis factor (TNF)-α) activates polymorphs, endothelium, platelets, complement and coagulation pathways. The activated white cells adhere to and damage vascular endothelium, allowing fluid and cells to leak into the interstitial space and microcirculatory thrombosis to impair tissue oxygen delivery. **Vasodilation** follows release of inflammatory mediators including nitric oxide (NO) from vascular endothelium. **Systolic and diastolic myocardial dysfunction** is due to reduced coronary perfusion and negative inotropic effects of NO and inflammatory mediators. **Impaired tissue oxygen utilization** is caused by sepsis-mediated cellular enzyme inhibition.

Clinical presentation

The clinical features of septic shock and potential sources of infection are illustrated in Figs a and c. Characteristic signs identify specific infections (e.g. splinter haemorrhages in endocarditis). The haemodynamic changes are variable (Chapter 4) and not related to the infecting organism. Circulatory assessment may reveal a hyperdynamic (i.e. 'warm, dilated') patient with bounding pulses. Alternatively, hypotension in a vasoconstricted (i.e. 'cold, clammy') septic patient can mimic pulmonary embolism or myocardial infarction. **Examination** may reveal a focus of infection or provide diagnostic clues (e.g. meningococcal rash). Chest infection is the commonest source of sepsis.

Management of severe sepsis
Identify and treat the cause (e.g. empyema drainage)
• **Essential investigations** include routine blood tests, C-reactive protein, plasma lactate, coagulation profile and arterial blood gases (ABG). **Cultures** of blood, sputum, urine and wound pus *must* be taken before starting antibiotics.
• **General investigations** include urinalysis, CXR and ECG.
• **Specific investigations** (Fig. c) depend on the suspected underlying cause (e.g. ultrasonography in intra-abdominal sepsis).
• **Antibiotic therapy** is initially *empirical* whilst microbiological results and sensitivities are awaited to guide therapy. The antibiotic regime is selected by determining the **most likely causative organisms**. This depends on clinical features, where the organism was contracted (i.e. community, hospital-acquired), the probable site of infection (i.e. chest) and local antibiotic resistance patterns. Risk factors for hospital-acquired infection include age, male sex, prolonged admission (>3 days), mechanical ventilation, trauma, catheters, drugs (e.g. steroids) and immunodeficiency.

General measures
• **General measures** include oxygen therapy, respiratory support, strict glycaemic control, nutrition and prophylaxis against stress ulceration and thromboembolism. **Monitor** vital signs, temperature, CVP (± cardiovascular monitoring), saturation, biochemical and ABG profiles.

Fluid, vasopressor and inotropic support (Chapter 5)
In **early septic shock**, widespread vasodilation causes hypotension and relative hypovolaemia. Associated reductions in LV afterload increase CO but inappropriate distribution can cause regional (e.g. splanchnic) ischaemia. Initially **fluid administration** corrects hypovolaemia, increases BP and restores organ perfusion. **As sepsis progresses**, toxic myocarditis impairs myocardial function, reducing CO and response to fluid administration. Excessive fluid may cause pulmonary oedema due to associated vascular permeability.
• **Vasopressor support** with noradrenaline, an α-vasoconstrictor agonist, increases SVR, BP and organ perfusion pressure without further fluid administration. However, CO may fall as SVR (afterload) increases if myocardial performance is impaired.
• **Inotropic support** (e.g. adrenaline, dopamine) increases cardiac contractility and maintains CO in these circumstances.

Additional measures
• **New therapies** include **activated protein C** which improves outcome in septic shock by modifying microcirculatory thrombosis and preventing organ ischaemia. Relative adrenocortical insufficiency is common in severe sepsis and **steroid therapy** is beneficial when hypotension is refractory to vasopressor support. **Anti-inflammatory therapies** (e.g. anti-TNF) are ineffective.
• **Sepsis prevention** includes infection control (e.g. hand washing), microbiological monitoring, prophylactic antibiotics for some invasive procedures and prompt management of suspected infection (e.g. early line changes).

Line-related sepsis
About 10–20% of central venous catheters (CVCs) become infected and associated sepsis is common. **Cause:** is usually non-sterile insertion technique or poor line care although infection from distant sites (e.g. endocarditis) or contamination from infusions (e.g. propofol) can occur. **Risk factors** are patient related (e.g. immunocompromise) or iatrogenic (e.g. emergency CVC insertion, prolonged catheterization, multilumen catheters). Femoral artery catheters are not at increased risk of contamination. Local inflammation and pus at the site of insertion are insensitive indicators of line infection. **Microbiology:** *S. aureus, S. epidermidis* and Gram-negative bacilli (e.g. *E. coli*) are the commonest organisms.
• **Management.** If line-related infection is suspected (i.e. sepsis ± positive blood cultures), the cannula is removed and the tip cultured. A new line is inserted at a different site. Empirical antibiotic therapy is started whilst awaiting microbiological results, although fever may resolve spontaneously after removal.
• **Prevention** of line infection requires strict aseptic insertion technique, firmly secured cannulae and closed systems. Avoid three-way tap contamination, give TPN through a dedicated lumen and change infusion sets regularly (e.g. 24–48h). The need for and timing of line replacement depend on whether the benefit outweighs the risks (e.g. pneumothorax). Scheduled replacement is not required, although probably change CVCs at 5–8 days.

17 End of life issues

(a) Brainstem death can only be diagnosed if all the following preconditions and exclusion criteria are met

Essential preconditions:
1) Apnoeic coma requiring ventilation
2) Irreversible brain damage due to an established cause

Factors that must be excluded:
a) Sedative drugs, neuromuscular blocking agents + poisons
 • Test blood and urine for drugs if doubt exists
b) Significant metabolic, acid-base or endocrine abnormalities:
 • metabolic (e.g. uraemia, hyponatraemia, liver encephalopathy)
 • acid-base (e.g. acidosis, CO_2 retention)
 • endocrine (e.g. diabetic, thyroid, Addisonian crisis)
c) Hypothermia (temperature <35 °C)
d) Severe hypotension

(b) Potential complications during the period before operative organ harvesting

Cardiovascular instability
 • hypotension; due to myocardial depression + vasodilation
 • autonomic instability; arrhythmias + bradycardia

Endocrine disorders
 • diabetes insipidus; diuresis, hypovolaemia, hypernatraemia
 • thyroid hormone deficiency
 • adrenal (cortisol) deficiency
 • pancreatic (insulin) deficiency; hyperglycaemia

Temperature control
 • hypothermia; due to ↓metabolic rate + ↓ muscle activity

Pulmonary oedema + hypoxaemia
Coagulopathy
Acid-base disorders + electrolyte imbalance

(c) Brainstem Function Testing: Criteria required to establish brain stem death (BSD) in the UK

The following 6 reflexes/responses must be absent to establish BSD

1. Pupillary responses:
Pupils must be fixed and unresponsive to light. Absent direct and consensual reactions confirm midbrain dysfunction. Pupillary size is irrelevant

2. Corneal reflex:
The reflex is absent if there is no blinking response to lightly touching the cornea with a piece of tissue paper

3. Vestibulo-ocular reflex (caloric testing): 30 mL of ice-cold water is slowly injected into each external auditory meatus after visualization of the ear-drums and removal of any obstructing wax

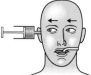 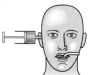

Normal reflex/response:
Conjugate eye deviation and nystagmus within ~20 s

Absent reflex:
no eye response. Confirms loss of pontine function

5. Motor response to painful stimuli:
Central (e.g. pressure between the eyes* or behind the ears**) or peripheral (e.g. limbs) painful stimuli cause no motor responses in cranial nerves. Normally grimacing occurs

6. Apnoea test:
Demonstrates absent respiratory effort despite a $PaCO_2$>6.7 kPa off the ventilator

After ventilation with 100% O_2 + whilst O_2 therapy is maintained through a tracheal catheter, the patient is disconnected from the ventilator and observed for respiratory effort. Apnoea confirms medullary dysfunction

Apnoea should continue until the $PaCO_2$ is >6.7 kPa on blood gas examination, which confirms adequate respiratory stimulation

Testing is discontinued if SaO_2 falls <90% or haemodynamic instability develops

4. 'Gag' and cough (tracheal) reflexes:
Pharyngeal/laryngeal stimulation (i.e. by endotracheal tube movement) normally causes 'gag'. Tracheal stimulation with a suction catheter normally causes cough. Absence of these reflexes indicates medullary dysfunction

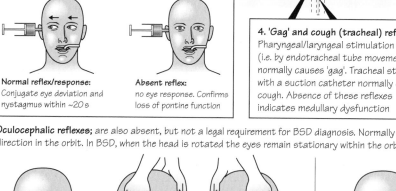

Oculocephalic reflexes; are also absent, but not a legal requirement for BSD diagnosis. Normally when the head is rotated the eyes move in the opposite direction in the orbit. In BSD, when the head is rotated the eyes remain stationary within the orbit (i.e move with the head)

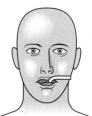 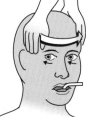 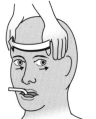 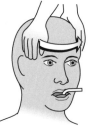 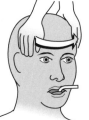 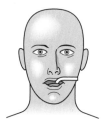

| Neutral head position | When head turned left | When head turned right | Neutral head position | If head is turned to the left or right, eyes do not |
| Eyes look forward | Eyes move rightwards | Eyes move leftwards | Eyes look forward | move in the orbit (i.e stare directly forwards) |

The normal oculocephalic reflex (eyes appear fixed on a distant object) | **Absent oculocephalic reflex (eyes appear immobile within the orbits)**

Critical care medicine is often life-saving and many patients make a complete recovery or achieve a quality of life (QOL) which, although impaired, is tolerable for the patient. However, treatment that prolongs the dying process or results in an unacceptable QOL may cause unnecessary suffering, loss of dignity and undue emotional distress. Unfortunately, in emergency situations, it is often impossible to identify those individuals who will not benefit from therapy. Consequently, following admission, humane and cost-effective management requires a willingness to withdraw or limit treatment when it becomes clear that the prognosis is poor. These decisions are often difficult and based on generally accepted **ethical and moral principles** including: (i) **beneficence**: the preservation of life, moderated by the need to relieve suffering; (ii) **non-maleficence or primum non nocere**: do no harm; (iii) **respect for autonomy**: the right to make informed choices; (iv) **justice**: fair allocation of medical resources; (v) **professional virtue** including compassion and integrity. The **'duty of care'** expected from medical professionals has been documented by statutory bodies including the British and American Medical Associations and the General Medical Council (UK).

Brainstem death

Brainstem death (BSD) is defined as irreversible loss of brainstem function with associated unconsciousness and cessation of spontaneous respiration. In the UK, BSD is considered to be a definition of death itself (i.e. despite a beating heart) as death due to cardiovascular failure always follows within ~1–21 days irrespective of mechanical ventilation. The purpose of establishing BSD is to demonstrate that continuing life-support is futile and to meet the legal requirements for organ donation (see below). The following criteria are used in the UK although there are international variations.

• **Diagnosis** requires that certain preconditions and exclusions are fulfilled (Fig. a).

• **Brainstem function tests (BSFTs)** are performed, >6–24 h after the precipitating event. Two doctors who are not part of the transplant team, one a consultant and both registered for >5 years, must complete two sets of BSFTs either separately or together. The six legally required findings that establish BSD are illustrated in Fig. (c). These are absent **pupillary, corneal, vestibulo-ocular** and **gag/cough reflexes, no cranial nerve motor responses** in response to painful stimuli, and **apnoea** following disconnection from the ventilator despite a $P_a\text{co}_2 > 6.7\,\text{kPa}$. Although not a legal requirement, **oculocephalic reflexes** are also absent. Seizure activity and decerebrate or decorticate posturing are inconsistent with BSD but spinal reflexes may occur. Some countries require an **EEG**, **radioisotope scan** or **cerebral angiography** to confirm BSD. Although there is no evidence that these increase diagnostic accuracy, they are useful when cranial nerve injuries or severe hypoxia prevents normal BSFTs.

Withdrawal of treatment (WOT)

The prognostic certainty of death associated with BSD relieves the anxiety associated with treatment discontinuation. However, when the brainstem is intact but cerebral cortex function ceases due to ischaemic damage (e.g. prolonged cardiac arrest) or diffuse cerebral injury (e.g. head trauma), spontaneous ventilation continues and prolonged survival without cognitive function is possi-

ble. This situation is termed **persistent vegetative state (PVS)**. In these patients, WOT decisions are difficult because there is often prognostic uncertainty. Previous ethical and medicolegal deliberations recommend that decision-making should focus on 'the likelihood of return to cognitive function' and that life-sustaining therapy should be withdrawn when it is clear that the patient is 'unlikely to regain cognitive behaviour, the ability to communicate or purposeful environmental interaction'. In these circumstances, it is generally agreed that treatment other than basic medical and nursing care is inappropriate. In **'severely disabled patients'** ethical dilemmas can be particularly complicated. It is important to appreciate that rational patients or legal surrogates have the right to refuse treatment even if this includes discontinuation of mechanical ventilation. Conversely, patients cannot demand life-saving therapy when clinicians consider it inappropriate. In practice, critically ill patients often cannot discuss treatment. Responsibility for WOT lies with the consultant or senior physician. Any such decisions made by other staff must be reviewed and confirmed by the consultant. Such judgements are always made in consultation with the family, taking into account prognosis, expected QOL, the opinions of the wider medical team (e.g. specialists, nursing staff) and the patient's previously expressed views (e.g. advance directives). It should be recognized that medical staff often underestimate a patient's willingness to undergo treatment independent of age or poor prognosis.

Once a WOT decision is made, **protocols** ensure patient comfort and dignity, reduce stress and reiterate the support required by relatives and junior staff. Physicians must decide which interventions to withdraw, recognizing that this will influence the rapidity, comfort and dignity of the patient's death. The usual preference for the order of WOT is: blood products, renal replacement therapy, inotropic support, antibiotics, mechanical ventilation, feeding and finally intravenous fluids. Unfortunately, these biases can prolong dying, causing unnecessary suffering. WOT plans must be regularly updated to prevent this. Narcotic or sedative therapy may be required to relieve discomfort, particularly when ventilation is discontinued.

Organ donation

Organ donation is a successful treatment for end-stage organ failure, limited only by the shortfall of organs for transplantation. Organ retrieval from suitable BSD patients must be maximized but dying patients should not be ventilated simply to allow organ donation. The question of organ donation is usually raised with relatives at the time of BSFT. The decision should be autonomous and 'unpressured'. The process is easier if the patient is a registered organ donor. Following consent, blood is sent for tissue typing, HIV, hepatitis and cytomegalovirus (CMV) testing. In the UK, each region has a transplant coordinator who, when contacted, will arrange retrieval and allocation of donated organs. Figure (b) lists **potential complications** prior to organ retrieval in the operating theatre. Graft survival is improved by maintaining preoperative organ perfusion (e.g. fluids, inotropes, monitoring) and oxygenation (i.e. $P_a\text{O}_2 > 10\,\text{kPa}$). Inotropes are selected to minimize organ dysfunction. Spinal reflexes and autonomic haemodynamic responses are controlled with neuromuscular blockers and opioids. Continuing emotional support for relatives and staff is essential.

18 Acute coronary syndromes

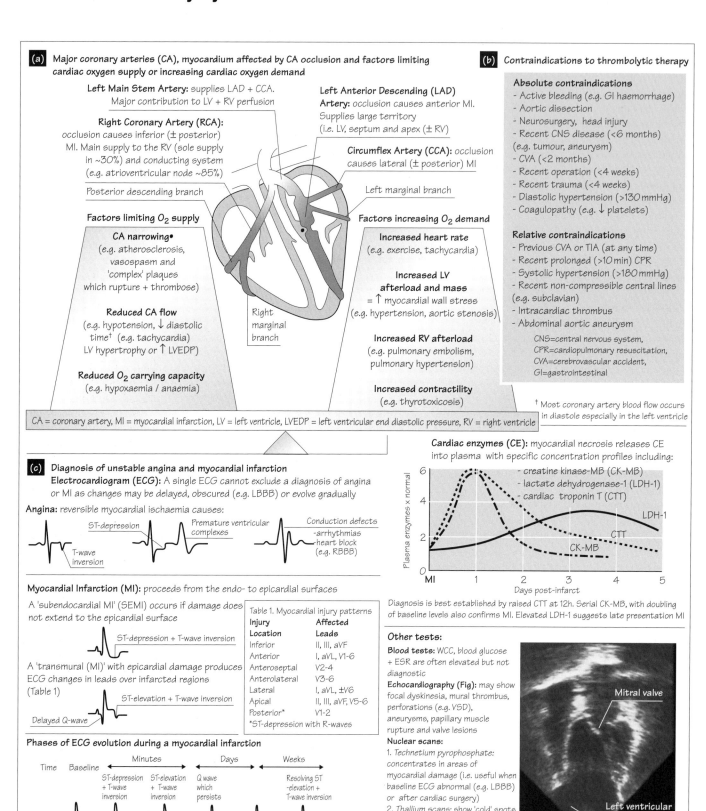

(a) Major coronary arteries (CA), myocardium affected by CA occlusion and factors limiting cardiac oxygen supply or increasing cardiac oxygen demand

Left Main Stem Artery: supplies LAD + CCA. Major contribution to LV + RV perfusion

Left Anterior Descending (LAD) Artery: occlusion causes anterior MI. Supplies large territory (i.e. LV, septum and apex (± RV)

Right Coronary Artery (RCA): occlusion causes inferior (± posterior) MI. Main supply to the RV (sole supply in ~30%) and conducting system (e.g. atrioventricular node ~85%)

Circumflex Artery (CCA): occlusion causes lateral (± posterior) MI

Posterior descending branch

Left marginal branch

Factors limiting O₂ supply

CA narrowing•
(e.g. atherosclerosis, vasospasm and 'complex' plaques which rupture + thrombose)

Reduced CA flow
(e.g. hypotension, ↓ diastolic time† (e.g. tachycardia) LV hypertrophy or ↑ LVEDP)

Reduced O₂ carrying capacity
(e.g. hypoxaemia / anaemia)

Right marginal branch

Factors increasing O₂ demand

Increased heart rate
(e.g. exercise, tachycardia)

Increased LV afterload and mass
= ↑ myocardial wall stress
(e.g. hypertension, aortic stenosis)

Increased RV afterload
(e.g. pulmonary embolism, pulmonary hypertension)

Increased contractility
(e.g. thyrotoxicosis)

CA = coronary artery, MI = myocardial infarction, LV = left ventricle, LVEDP = left ventricular end diastolic pressure, RV = right ventricle

(b) Contraindications to thrombolytic therapy

Absolute contraindications
- Active bleeding (e.g. GI haemorrhage)
- Aortic dissection
- Neurosurgery, head injury
- Recent CNS disease (<6 months) (e.g. tumour, aneurysm)
- CVA (<2 months)
- Recent operation (<4 weeks)
- Recent trauma (<4 weeks)
- Diastolic hypertension (>130 mmHg)
- Coagulopathy (e.g. ↓ platelets)

Relative contraindications
- Previous CVA or TIA (at any time)
- Recent prolonged (>10 min) CPR
- Systolic hypertension (>180 mmHg)
- Recent non-compressible central lines (e.g. subclavian)
- Intracardiac thrombus
- Abdominal aortic aneurysm

CNS=central nervous system,
CPR=cardiopulmonary resuscitation,
CVA=cerebrovascular accident,
GI=gastrointestinal

† Most coronary artery blood flow occurs in diastole especially in the left ventricle

(c) Diagnosis of unstable angina and myocardial infarction
Electrocardiogram (ECG): A single ECG cannot exclude a diagnosis of angina or MI as changes may be delayed, obscured (e.g. LBBB) or evolve gradually

Angina: reversible myocardial ischaemia causes:

ST-depression

T-wave inversion

Premature ventricular complexes

Conduction defects
-arrhythmias
-heart block
(e.g. RBBB)

Cardiac enzymes (CE): myocardial necrosis releases CE into plasma with specific concentration profiles including:
- creatine kinase-MB (CK-MB)
- lactate dehydrogenase-1 (LDH-1)
- cardiac troponin T (CTT)

Diagnosis is best established by raised CTT at 12h. Serial CK-MB, with doubling of baseline levels also confirms MI. Elevated LDH-1 suggests late presentation MI

Myocardial Infarction (MI): proceeds from the endo- to epicardial surfaces

A 'subendocardial MI' (SEMI) occurs if damage does not extend to the epicardial surface

ST-depression + T-wave inversion

A 'transmural (MI)' with epicardial damage produces ECG changes in leads over infarcted regions (Table 1)

ST-elevation + T-wave inversion

Delayed Q-wave

Table 1. Myocardial injury patterns

Injury Location	Affected Leads
Inferior	II, III, aVF
Anterior	I, aVL, V1-6
Anteroseptal	V2-4
Anterolateral	V3-6
Lateral	I, aVL, ±V6
Apical	II, III, aVF, V5-6
Posterior*	V1-2

*ST-depression with R-waves

Other tests:

Blood tests: WCC, blood glucose + ESR are often elevated but not diagnostic

Echocardiography (Fig): may show focal dyskinesia, mural thrombus, perforations (e.g. VSD), aneurysms, papillary muscle rupture and valve lesions

Nuclear scans:
1. Technetium pyrophosphate: concentrates in areas of myocardial damage (i.e. useful when baseline ECG abnormal (e.g. LBBB) or after cardiac surgery)
2. Thallium scans: show 'cold' spots in non-perfused myocardium and demonstrate areas of reversible ischaemia

Mitral valve

Left ventricular aneurysm

Phases of ECG evolution during a myocardial infarction

Time	Baseline	Minutes		Days	Weeks
		ST-depression + T-wave inversion	ST-elevation + T-wave inversion	Q wave which persists	Resolving ST -elevation + T-wave inversion
ECG	Normal	Ischaemia or SEMI	Myocardial Damage	Recovery	

ESR = erythrocyte sedimentation rate, LBBB= left bundle branch block, RBBB = right bundle branch block, VSD = ventricular septal defect, WCC = white cell count

Epidemiology

Ischaemic heart disease is the main cause of death in developed countries, causing ~30% of male and ~20% of female deaths in the UK. **Incidence** increases with age, male sex and post-menopause in women. **Risk factors** include hypertension, hypercholesterolaemia, cigarette smoking, family history and diabetes mellitus. **Myocardial infarction** (MI) occurs in ~300 000 people annually in the UK and ~140 000 die; 33–66% of deaths occur before hospital admission, ~10–15% after admission and ~20–30% within 2 years due to heart failure or further MI.

Pathogenesis

Myocardial ischaemia results from an imbalance between oxygen supply and demand (Fig. a). Coronary artery (CA) narrowing by smooth, 'occlusive' atherosclerotic plaques without overlying thrombosis causes **stable angina** (SA). Small, non-occlusive (i.e <50% CA narrowing) 'complex' plaques with lipid-rich cores and thin fibrous caps can rupture under stress (e.g. hypertension) causing overlying subocclusive thrombus, vasospasm and **unstable angina** (UA). If untreated, UA can progress to MI or sudden cardiac death (~15–30%) within weeks. **Myocardial infarction** is due to fresh occlusive CA thrombus overlying atherosclerotic lesions in ~90% at angiography. MI with normal CA is rare (<10%) but may follow embolic occlusion (e.g. endocarditis), non-thrombotic vasospasm or cocaine abuse.

Clinical features

Myocardial ischaemia causes 'crushing' or heavy substernal chest pain radiating to the neck and medial aspect of the left arm which is usually more severe in MI than angina. Pain may be atypical (e.g. burning), localized (e.g. jaw only) or absent in ~20% (e.g. diabetics). **SA** is usually precipitated by exercise or anxiety, is short-lived and is relieved by rest and sublingual nitrates. **UA** occurs at rest, more frequently and for longer periods (>15 min) than SA. 'New pain', 'altered SA pattern' (i.e. with less exercise), autonomic manifestations (e.g. nausea, sweating) and radiation to new sites (e.g. jaw, arm) also suggest UA.

MI is characterized by abrupt onset of severe, prolonged pain, autonomic symptoms, dyspnoea and anxiety. UA only precedes MI in ~25% of cases. Tachycardia accompanies anterior MI whereas bradycardia (±heart block) is more frequent after inferior MI (i.e. conducting tissue damage). Hypotension (systolic BP < 90 mmHg) suggests a large MI (>40% LV damage) and heralds cardiogenic shock (Chapters 4, 5). Auscultation often reveals a fourth heart sound and gallop rhythm.

- **MI complications** include arrhythmias (Chapter 19), papillary muscle or free wall rupture, pericarditis and ventricular septal defects. Heart failure may occur with >20% LV damage.
- **Investigations.** Serial ECGs and **cardiac enzymes** establish the diagnosis (Fig. c). A raised **cardiac troponin T** (CTT) is particularly useful to confirm MI after surgery or when the ECG is non-specific (>40% MIs are non-Q wave). In **non-MI acute coronary syndrome**s (e.g. UA) a raised CTT indicates an increased risk of subsequent MI.

UA management

Management of UA aims to relieve symptoms and prevent MI.
- **Antianginal therapy** *reduces myocardial oxygen consumption (MOC)* by lowering heart rate (e.g. bed rest, β-blockers) and afterload (e.g. antihypertensives) and *increases myocardial oxygen supply* using oxygen and pharmacotherapy. **Nitrates** dilate CA and decrease LV wall tension by reducing preload and to a lesser degree afterload. Sublingual, oral and intravenous routes are rapidly effective. **Slow calcium channel blockers** (e.g. nifedipine) relieve CA vasospasm but are negatively inotropic and cause detrimental tachycardia.
- **Antithrombotic therapy.** Within 15 min of chewing non-enteric **aspirin** tablets, irreversible COX inhibition prevents platelet aggregation, reducing the risk of MI and death by 50%. Antiplatelet agents, which inhibit glycoprotein IIb/IIIa, are useful in patients with aspirin allergy but onset of action is slow. Intravenous **heparin**, in combination with aspirin, further reduces morbidity and mortality. Dipyridamole does not enhance aspirin effects. **Thrombolytics** *do not* reduce MI or mortality in UA.
- **Early revascularization (e.g. angioplasty)** does not improve outcome but is considered after 48 h if medical therapy fails.

MI management

Early reperfusion and minimizing MOC limit infarct size and reduce hospital mortality from 30% to <10%.
- **Acute management** includes bed rest, cardiac monitoring (~48 h) and >60% oxygen. Immediate **aspirin** prevents further platelet aggregation. Sublingual **nitrates** reduce pain, MOC and infarct size but may aggravate hypotension. **Opiates** (e.g. diamorphine) relieve pain and reduce MOC by decreasing preload and catecholamine release. Early **β-blockade** (e.g. metoprolol) limits infarct size, arrhythmias and mortality but contraindications include asthma, heart failure and bradycardia. Oral **ACE inhibitors**, started 24 h after admission, improve LV remodelling and reduce heart failure in high-risk patients. Unless contraindicated, prophylactic **subcutaneous heparin** prevents thromboembolic complications. The value of prophylactic anti-arrhythmic therapy is not established. Cardiogenic shock and **inotropic support** are discussed in Chapters 4 and 5.
- **Thrombolytic therapy (TT)** breaks down CA clot, reperfuses ischaemic tissue, limits myocardial damage and reduces complications (e.g. heart failure). Mortality falls by >25% if TT is given within 12 h but is most effective within 3 h. Reperfusion occurs in 50–75% of cases. TT accelerates conversion of plasminogen to plasmin, an enzyme that attacks fibrin. Consequently, it increases the risk of haemorrhage and contraindications (Fig. b) prevent use in ~50% of cases. **Streptokinase** (SK) is allergenic and can only be used once; ~2% have reactions with first use. **Tissue plasminogen activator** (TPA) only activates plasminogen bound to fibrin (i.e. better targeted at thrombus). If given within 3 h, it is more effective than SK but surprisingly causes more strokes. TPA is given if SK has been used previously. Intravenous heparin is required for 48–72 h after TPA.
- **Percutaneous coronary angioplasty (PTCA)** is limited by availability. Primary PTCA (i.e. within <6 h and instead of TT) reopens >90% of occluded CAs with few complications. Rescue PTCA is considered if TT fails, but mortality is ~40% if unsuccessful.
- **Ongoing management.** Reduce risk factors (e.g. smoking). Patients with UA or at high risk on exercise testing are referred for angiography and early revascularization. **Warfarin** is administered for 3 months after large infarctions, aspirin is continued indefinitely, but β-blockers and ACE inhibitors may be discontinued after 6–52 weeks in low-risk patients.

19 Arrhythmias

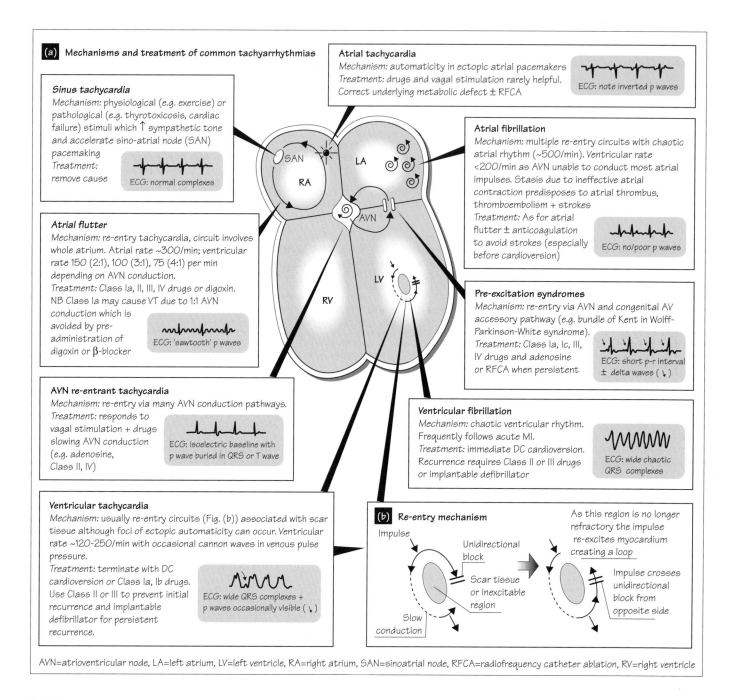

(a) Mechanisms and treatment of common tachyarrhythmias

Sinus tachycardia
Mechanism: physiological (e.g. exercise) or pathological (e.g. thyrotoxicosis, cardiac failure) stimuli which ↑ sympathetic tone and accelerate sino-atrial node (SAN) pacemaking
Treatment: remove cause
ECG: normal complexes

Atrial tachycardia
Mechanism: automaticity in ectopic atrial pacemakers
Treatment: drugs and vagal stimulation rarely helpful. Correct underlying metabolic defect ± RFCA
ECG: note inverted p waves

Atrial fibrillation
Mechanism: multiple re-entry circuits with chaotic atrial rhythm (~500/min). Ventricular rate <200/min as AVN unable to conduct most atrial impulses. Stasis due to ineffective atrial contraction predisposes to atrial thrombus, thromboembolism + strokes
Treatment: As for atrial flutter ± anticoagulation to avoid strokes (especially before cardioversion)
ECG: no/poor p waves

Atrial flutter
Mechanism: re-entry tachycardia, circuit involves whole atrium. Atrial rate ~300/min; ventricular rate 150 (2:1), 100 (3:1), 75 (4:1) per min depending on AVN conduction.
Treatment: Class Ia, II, III, IV drugs or digoxin. NB Class Ia may cause VT due to 1:1 AVN conduction which is avoided by pre-administration of digoxin or β-blocker
ECG: 'sawtooth' p waves

Pre-excitation syndromes
Mechanism: re-entry via AVN and congenital AV accessory pathway (e.g. bundle of Kent in Wolff-Parkinson-White syndrome).
Treatment: Class Ia, Ic, III, IV drugs and adenosine or RFCA when persistent
ECG: short p-r interval ± delta waves (↘)

AVN re-entrant tachycardia
Mechanism: re-entry via many AVN conduction pathways.
Treatment: responds to vagal stimulation + drugs slowing AVN conduction (e.g. adenosine, Class II, IV)
ECG: Isoelectric baseline with p wave buried in QRS or T wave

Ventricular fibrillation
Mechanism: chaotic ventricular rhythm. Frequently follows acute MI.
Treatment: immediate DC cardioversion. Recurrence requires Class II or III drugs or implantable defibrillator
ECG: wide chaotic QRS complexes

Ventricular tachycardia
Mechanism: usually re-entry circuits (Fig. (b)) associated with scar tissue although foci of ectopic automaticity can occur. Ventricular rate ~120-250/min with occasional cannon waves in venous pulse pressure.
Treatment: terminate with DC cardioversion or Class Ia, Ib drugs. Use Class II or III to prevent initial recurrence and implantable defibrillator for persistent recurrence.
ECG: wide QRS complexes + p waves occasionally visible (↘)

(b) Re-entry mechanism
Impulse
Unidirectional block
Scar tissue or inexcitable region
Slow conduction
As this region is no longer refractory the impulse re-excites myocardium creating a loop
Impulse crosses unidirectional block from opposite side

AVN=atrioventricular node, LA=left atrium, LV=left ventricle, RA=right atrium, SAN=sinoatrial node, RFCA=radiofrequency catheter ablation, RV=right ventricle

Definition
Arrhythmias are abnormalities of the heart rate (HR) or rhythm. **Tachycardia** is an HR > 100 beats/min and is supraventricular (SVT) or ventricular (VT) in origin. Tachycardias are caused by:
1 *Increased pacemaker activity*. Faster spontaneous membrane depolarization, lower thresholds or oscillations during repolarization (e.g. digoxin toxicity) trigger early action potentials (APs).
2 *Re-entry circuits*. A wave of depolarization travels in a circle of myocardial tissue; provided tissue is not refractory when the electrical impulse returns, it will depolarize again producing a recurring circuit (Fig. b). This causes most paroxysmal tachycardias.

Bradycardia is an HR <60 beats/min and is due to abnormal and delayed cardiac conduction.

General management
Arrhythmias are common in critically ill patients. They must be rapidly assessed (i.e. clinical response), diagnosed and treated. **Prevention** requires early correction of hypoxaemia, electrolyte disturbances (e.g. hypokalaemia, hypomagnesaemia), acid–base imbalance and cardiac ischaemia. Arrhythmogenic factors including pain, vagal stimulation (e.g. suctioning), drugs (e.g. theophylline) and cardiac irritants (e.g. intracardiac catheters) must be

addressed. **Tachyarrhythmias** are detrimental when they cause symptoms (e.g. dizziness) or reduce tissue perfusion. They are terminated immediately with cardioversion (±drugs) if causing hypotension, pulmonary oedema or angina (Chapter 21). **Bradyarrhythmias**, if symptomatic, are treated with atropine, β-agonists or pacing (see below). *Not all arrhythmias require intervention*; those that are asymptomatic or stable are observed whilst the cause (e.g. electrolyte imbalance) is corrected.

- **Vagal stimulation** (e.g. carotid sinus massage) slows HR, allowing precise diagnosis and may cardiovert some SVTs.
- **Antiarrhythmic drugs** are classified by mechanism or site of action (above and Appendix, p. 106). They are selected according to rhythm and underlying pathophysiology (Fig. a). Therapeutic windows are often narrow, side-effects common (e.g. CNS), therapy is frequently ineffective (e.g. ~50% of serious VT) and paradoxically they cause new arrhythmias in ~20% of patients. **'Proarrhythmic' effects** are common with Class Ia and III drugs which increase AP duration (i.e. prolonged QT interval), trigger automaticity and precipitate dangerous VT (e.g. 'torsades de pointes'). **Prophylaxis:** Arrhythmia suppression does not always improve outcome (e.g. lignocaine after myocardial infarction) although β-blockers reduce mortality in IHD.
- **Non-pharmacological therapies** may be required in emergency situations and can be more successful than protracted drug therapy. In haemodynamically unstable VT or SVT, **direct current (DC) cardioversion** using 50–360-J shocks delivered through electrodes placed over the sternum and cardiac apex in anaesthetized patients achieves rapid cardioversion (Chapter 21). In patients with recurrent VT, **implantable defibrillators** improve survival by >30% compared to drug therapy. **Radiofrequency catheter ablation** (RFCA) safely eliminates >90% of treatable accessory pathways or ectopic pacemaker lesions using localized heat delivered through a catheter tip. In refractory SVT **overdrive atrial pacing** may restore sinus rhythm.

Diagnosis

Arrhythmia diagnosis may be difficult. Interpretation of ECG or rhythm strips can be complicated by electrical artifacts, shivering, seizure activity and tremors. Occasionally specialized oesophageal or right-sided ECG leads aid diagnosis.
- **Narrow QRS complex (NC) tachycardias** are usually due to SVT and can be assessed (and terminated) with intravenous adenosine boluses.
- **Wide QRS complex (WC) tachycardias** are usually due to VT but can be difficult to differentiate from SVT with abnormal conduction (SVT/AC). Treat as VT if haemodynamic instability coexists after excluding atrioventricular node (AVN) block. Lack of response to cardioversion and/or intravenous lignocaine suggests an SVT/AC which may be confirmed and cardioverted with adenosine. Further failure to respond is managed with repeated cardioversion and intravenous amiodarone which slows HR and improves haemodynamic stability (Appendix, p. 106).

Tachyarrhythmias

Mechanisms and treatments are summarized in Fig. (a).

1 *Supraventricular tachyarrhythmias* originate above the AVN and present with dizziness, palpitations and breathlessness. They are rarely life-threatening, although sudden death can occur.
- **Sinus tachycardia,** the commonest SVT, is a normal physiological response to stress.
- **Atrial tachycardias** are due to ectopic atrial automaticity in chronic heart and lung disease with associated metabolic, acid–base or drug (e.g. digoxin, theophylline) toxicity.
- **Atrial flutter** and **fibrillation** may occur in isolation but are commonly associated with cardiac disease (e.g. atrial dilation, hypertension), thyrotoxicosis or thromboembolism.
- **AVN re-entrant tachycardia** is common, whereas **pre-excitation syndromes** are unusual causes of SVT.

2 *Ventricular tachyarrhythmias* usually arise in the ventricles of patients with underlying IHD, cardiomyopathy or congenital heart disease. They are generally more serious than SVT.
- **Ventricular tachycardia** is occasionally well tolerated but often causes haemodynamic instability or degenerates into **ventricular fibrillation (VF)** with immediate loss of CO and unconsciousness. Death follows without resuscitation and DC cardioversion (Chapter 21).

Bradyarrhythmias

Bradyarrhythmias are well tolerated by normal hearts. However, CO and BP fall if stroke volume cannot increase due to reduced cardiac compliance or contractility.

1 *Sinus bradycardia* has normal ECG p-waves and 1:1 AVN conduction. Correction of potential causes including vagal reflexes (e.g. pain, hypoxaemia), drug toxicity (e.g. β-blockers) or AVN ischaemia is usually remedial. Treatment with atropine, β-agonists (e.g. isoprenaline) or drug antidotes (e.g. digoxin antibodies) may be required if symptoms persist.

2 *Heart block (HB)* is usually due to ischaemic damage to nodal or conducting tissue. Although common after inferior MI, because the right coronary artery supplies the AVN, it is transient and rarely requires intervention. In contrast, HB after anterior MI suggests a large infarct and requires early pacemaker insertion.
- **First-degree HB** slows AVN conduction causing p–r prolongation (>0.2s) on ECG. It is unimportant except as an early warning of higher degrees of HB.
- **Second-degree HB** occurs when some atrial beats are not conducted to the ventricles.

  Mobitz I AVN block (Wenckebach) causes p–r interval lengthening, culminating in failure of transmission of an atrial impulse. This sequence is repetitive. Treatment is rarely required.

  Mobitz II block originates below the AVN in the His–Purkinje system. Every second or third atrial impulse initiates ventricular contraction (2:1; 3:1 block). Pacemaker insertion may be required (e.g. anterior MI) as complete HB can develop.
- In **complete (third-degree) HB**, conduction between atria and ventricles ceases.

  AVN pacemaker activity produces NC 'junctional rhythms' (HR ~40–60 beats/min), which are often transient and asymptomatic.

  Infranodal WC pacemaker activity is unstable, slower (HR ~30–45 beats/min) and symptomatic. A pacemaker is essential.

20 Heart failure and pulmonary oedema

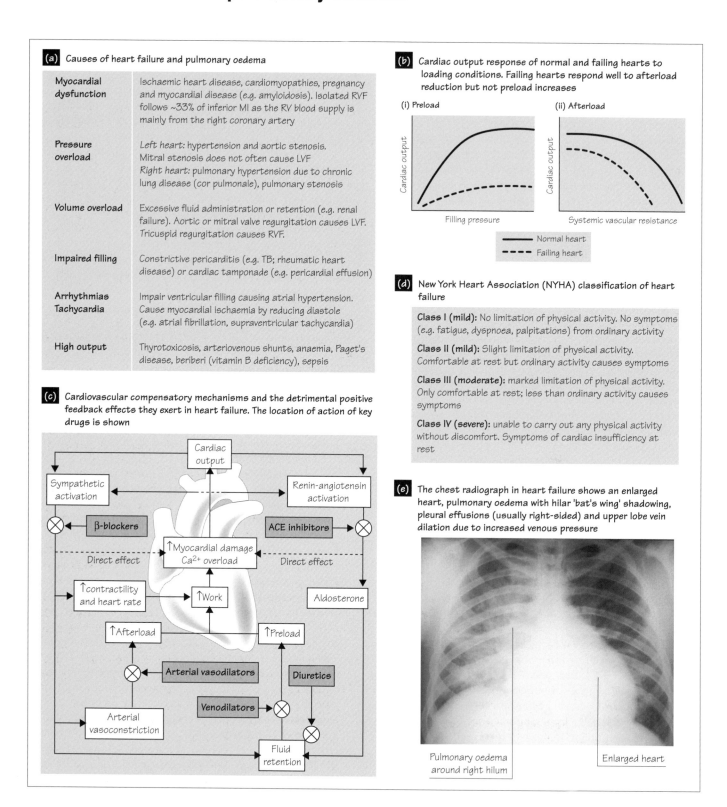

(a) Causes of heart failure and pulmonary oedema

Myocardial dysfunction	Ischaemic heart disease, cardiomyopathies, pregnancy and myocardial disease (e.g. amyloidosis). Isolated RVF follows ~33% of inferior MI as the RV blood supply is mainly from the right coronary artery
Pressure overload	Left heart: hypertension and aortic stenosis. Mitral stenosis does not often cause LVF. Right heart: pulmonary hypertension due to chronic lung disease (cor pulmonale), pulmonary stenosis
Volume overload	Excessive fluid administration or retention (e.g. renal failure). Aortic or mitral valve regurgitation causes LVF. Tricuspid regurgitation causes RVF.
Impaired filling	Constrictive pericarditis (e.g. TB; rheumatic heart disease) or cardiac tamponade (e.g. pericardial effusion)
Arrhythmias Tachycardia	Impair ventricular filling causing atrial hypertension. Cause myocardial ischaemia by reducing diastole (e.g. atrial fibrillation, supraventricular tachycardia)
High output	Thyrotoxicosis, arteriovenous shunts, anaemia, Paget's disease, beriberi (vitamin B deficiency), sepsis

(b) Cardiac output response of normal and failing hearts to loading conditions. Failing hearts respond well to afterload reduction but not preload increases

(i) Preload — Cardiac output vs Filling pressure

(ii) Afterload — Cardiac output vs Systemic vascular resistance

—— Normal heart
- - - Failing heart

(c) Cardiovascular compensatory mechanisms and the detrimental positive feedback effects they exert in heart failure. The location of action of key drugs is shown

(d) New York Heart Association (NYHA) classification of heart failure

Class I (mild): No limitation of physical activity. No symptoms (e.g. fatigue, dyspnoea, palpitations) from ordinary activity

Class II (mild): Slight limitation of physical activity. Comfortable at rest but ordinary activity causes symptoms

Class III (moderate): marked limitation of physical activity. Only comfortable at rest; less than ordinary activity causes symptoms

Class IV (severe): unable to carry out any physical activity without discomfort. Symptoms of cardiac insufficiency at rest

(e) The chest radiograph in heart failure shows an enlarged heart, pulmonary oedema with hilar 'bat's wing' shadowing, pleural effusions (usually right-sided) and upper lobe vein dilation due to increased venous pressure

Pulmonary oedema around right hilum

Enlarged heart

Normal cardiac output (CO) is ~5 L/min and >25 L/min during exercise. **Heart failure** (HF) occurs when the heart cannot maintain adequate CO to perfuse the tissues, or does so only with elevated filling pressures (Chapters 4, 5). Consequently, HF may limit exercise tolerance, increase 'downstream' hydrostatic pressure or reduce CO. The left, right or both sides of the heart can fail.

- **Left ventricular failure** (LVF) is most common. If the resulting 'downstream' pulmonary capillary ('wedge') pressure (PCWP; Chapters 2, 4) rises to >20–25 mmHg, fluid filters into alveolar and interstitial spaces causing **pulmonary oedema** and congestion (e.g. pleural effusions). Pulmonary oedema develops at lower PCWP when plasma oncotic pressure falls (e.g. hypoalbuminaemia) or membrane permeability increases (e.g. inflammation).
- **Right ventricular failure** (RVF) causes systemic congestion (e.g. ankle oedema) and is usually due to LVF. Resulting biventricular failure is termed **congestive cardiac failure** (CCF).
- '**Cor pulmonale**' describes RVF due to chronic lung disease.

Epidemiology

HF affects 2–3% of the population and >10% of people >75 years old. In developed countries it is commoner in men. **Causes** are listed in Fig. (a); the most common is IHD. However, pulmonary oedema may occur despite good contractile function (e.g. volume overload). **Prognosis:** The 5-year survival is ~50%.

Pathophysiology

- **Systolic (contractile) dysfunction** is usually due to IHD, although cardiomyopathy, toxicity (e.g. metabolic), valve defects and arrhythmias also reduce ventricular ejection fraction and contractility. Initially CO is maintained by compensatory mechanisms including: (i) *increased sympathetic drive*; (ii) *raised circulating volume* (i.e. salt and water retention due to activation of the renin–angiotensin system by poor renal perfusion); (iii) *raised filling pressures* (Fig. b(i); Chapters 4, 5). Unfortunately, these mechanisms also have detrimental effects: failing hearts respond poorly to preload (Fig. b(i)) with subsequent pulmonary and peripheral congestion, whilst large ventricular volumes increase cardiac work, reduce efficiency and further impair function (Fig. c). In pressure overload (e.g. aortic stenosis), compensatory hypertrophy initially assists ventricular ejection but reduced capillary density and compliance eventually decrease blood supply and contractility.
- **Diastolic (relaxation) dysfunction** (DD) occurs when LV relaxation, an energy-dependent process, is impaired. Myocardial ischaemia due to IHD or LV hypertrophy (e.g. hypertension) with poor diastolic LV perfusion is the commonest cause. Reduced LV compliance decreases filling and may precipitate pulmonary oedema despite normal contractility. DD affects ~33% of HF patients and may be precipitated by tachycardia (shorter diastolic perfusion time) or atrial fibrillation (impaired LV filling).

Clinical features

Clinical features depend on speed of onset, underlying cause and ventricular involvement. HF can be precipitated or aggravated by many factors (e.g. pregnancy). Whatever the cause, low CO causes fatigue, anorexia and exercise limitation, with severity defined by the **New York Heart Association (NYHA) classification** (Fig. d). **LVF** is characterized by breathlessness, hypoxaemia, orthopnoea, paroxysmal nocturnal dyspnoea and cough productive of frothy 'pink' sputum. Auscultation may reveal a gallop rhythm (S_3/S_4 added sounds) and coarse crepitations at the lung bases. **RVF** causes systemic congestion with raised jugular venous pressure, hepatomegaly, ascites and ankle oedema. Onset may be **acute** (e.g. MI) with cardiogenic shock (Chapter 4) or acute pulmonary oedema, or **chronic** with fatigue and gradual fluid retention.

Diagnostic investigations

Investigations include cardiac enzymes, ECG and chest radiography (Fig. e). Echocardiography may demonstrate wall hypokinesia and ventricular enlargement. Ejection fraction is always reduced although CO and BP may be normal (see above).

Management

Management must address the cause (e.g. IHD, valve disease), underlying pathophysiology (e.g. DD) and precipitating events (e.g. arrhythmias). In general, **afterload reduction** rapidly improves LV function and CO in the failing heart (Fig. b(ii)) but may cause hypotension. In contrast, **preload reduction** relieves symptoms (e.g. pulmonary oedema) but CO is not increased (Fig. b(i)), except when afterload is indirectly reduced (e.g. decreased chamber size). **Non-invasive monitoring** (e.g. PiCCO) and less frequently **pulmonary artery catheterization** may be required to measure filling pressures, CO and vascular resistances to optimize HF treatment (Chapters 2, 4, 5).

- **Acute left ventricular failure.** The immediate priority is relief of breathlessness due to pulmonary oedema. The **sitting position** is most comfortable and **supplemental oxygen** (>60%) corrects hypoxaemia. Intravenous **loop diuretics** (e.g. furosemide) cause pulmonary venodilation, reduce LV preload and relieve dyspnoea. Subsequent diuresis lowers fluid load and cardiac filling pressures. Intravenous **nitrates** also increase venous capacitance whilst simultaneously dilating coronary arteries in IHD. **Diamorphine** decreases preload due to potent venodilator effects. It also relieves anxiety, thereby reducing Vo_2. **Bronchodilators** (e.g. salbutamol) reverse bronchospasm but aminophylline may precipitate arrhythmias. **CPAP** is used with increasing frequency in HF (Chapter 8) and rapidly reduces hypoxaemia and work of breathing. **Arrhythmia** correction is essential (Chapter 19).
- **Low-output left ventricular failure.** When pulmonary oedema has been controlled, treatment aims to improve LV function, DD and prognosis. **ACE inhibitors** reduce afterload, increase CO, reduce symptoms (e.g. fatigue) and lengthen survival. They benefit most patients with HF except when contraindicated (e.g. renal artery stenosis) or if side-effects occur (e.g. cough). Selective β-**blockers** (e.g. carvedilol) improve prognosis by reducing myocardial ischaemia and arrhythmias but may precipitate pulmonary oedema, heart block or bronchospasm. **Calcium channel blockers (CCBs)** alleviate DD by reducing hypertension and coronary vasospasm. However, simultaneous tachycardia and impaired cardiac contractility limit use. **Digoxin** has transient inotropic effects and is of particular value in HF with AF. **Prophylactic anticoagulants** reduce associated thromboembolic events.
- **Right ventricular failure.** Diuresis reduces systemic oedema but is detrimental if high RV filling pressures are required to maintain CO. Systemic hypotension usually limits benefit from afterload reduction with pulmonary vasodilators (e.g. CCBs). **Oxygen therapy** relieves cor pulmonale (Chapter 25).
- **Cardiogenic shock** is discussed in Chapters 4 and 5. **Inotropic agents** or **intra-aortic balloon pumps** are often required to maintain CO and perfusion pressures. **Phosphodiesterase inhibitors** (milrinone) increase cAMP, stimulating cardiac contractility and peripheral vasodilation. Similarly, new **calcium sensitizers** may enhance contractility. Early **ventilatory support** may improve survival (Chapters 8, 10).

21 Cardiopulmonary resuscitation

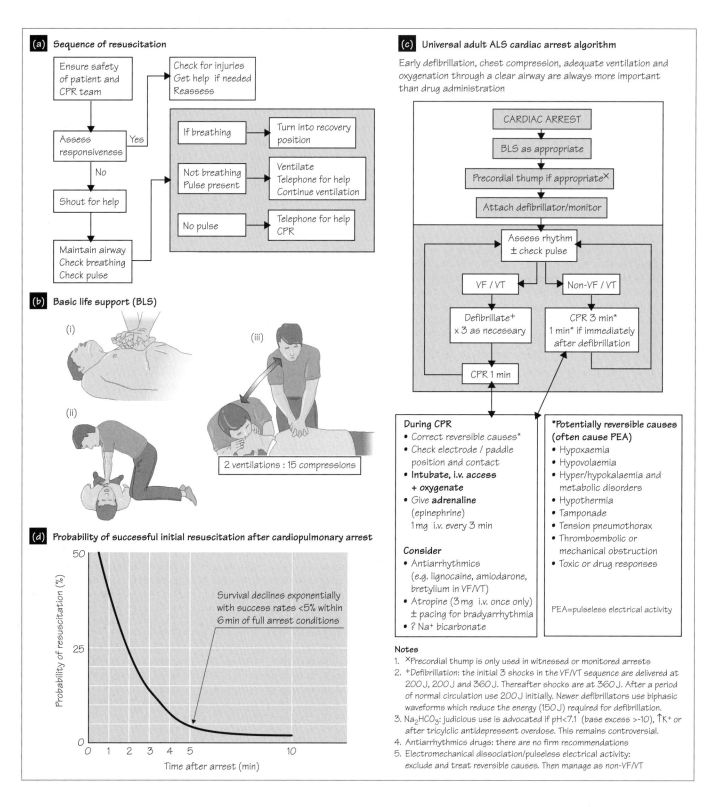

(a) Sequence of resuscitation

Ensure safety of patient and CPR team → Check for injuries / Get help if needed / Reassess

Assess responsiveness — Yes →
Shout for help
Maintain airway / Check breathing / Check pulse

If breathing → Turn into recovery position

Not breathing / Pulse present → Ventilate / Telephone for help / Continue ventilation

No pulse → Telephone for help / CPR

(b) Basic life support (BLS)

(i)
(ii)
(iii)

2 ventilations : 15 compressions

(c) Universal adult ALS cardiac arrest algorithm

Early defibrillation, chest compression, adequate ventilation and oxygenation through a clear airway are always more important than drug administration

CARDIAC ARREST
BLS as appropriate
Precordial thump if appropriate×
Attach defibrillator/monitor
Assess rhythm ± check pulse
VF / VT | Non-VF / VT
Defibrillate+ x 3 as necessary | CPR 3 min* / 1 min* if immediately after defibrillation
CPR 1 min

During CPR
- Correct reversible causes*
- Check electrode / paddle position and contact
- **Intubate, i.v. access + oxygenate**
- Give **adrenaline** (epinephrine) 1 mg i.v. every 3 min

Consider
- Antiarrhythmics (e.g. lignocaine, amiodarone, bretylium in VF/VT)
- Atropine (3 mg i.v. once only) ± pacing for bradyarrhythmia
- ? Na+ bicarbonate

*Potentially reversible causes (often cause PEA)
- Hypoxaemia
- Hypovolaemia
- Hyper/hypokalaemia and metabolic disorders
- Hypothermia
- Tamponade
- Tension pneumothorax
- Thromboembolic or mechanical obstruction
- Toxic or drug responses

PEA=pulseless electrical activity

Notes
1. ×Precordial thump is only used in witnessed or monitored arrests
2. +Defibrillation: the initial 3 shocks in the VF/VT sequence are delivered at 200 J, 200 J and 360 J. Thereafter shocks are at 360 J. After a period of normal circulation use 200 J initially. Newer defibrillators use biphasic waveforms which reduce the energy (150 J) required for defibrillation.
3. Na_2HCO_3: judicious use is advocated if pH<7.1 (base excess >-10), ↑K+ or after tricylclic antidepressent overdose. This remains controversial.
4. Antiarrhythmics drugs: there are no firm recommendations
5. Electromechanical dissociation/pulseless electrical activity: exclude and treat reversible causes. Then manage as non-VF/VT

(d) Probability of successful initial resuscitation after cardiopulmonary arrest

Survival declines exponentially with success rates <5% within 6 min of full arrest conditions

(y-axis: Probability of resuscitation (%), 0 to 50)
(x-axis: Time after arrest (min), 0 to 10)

Cardiopulmonary arrests (CPAs) are cardiac or respiratory in origin. Cardiopulmonary resuscitation (CPR) aims to preserve neurological function by rapidly restoring oxygenation, ventilation and circulation during circulatory and/or ventilatory arrest. Most

out-of-hospital arrests (OHAs) are due to IHD and in ~80% the preterminal arrhythmia is VF. In contrast, ~50% of in-hospital arrests (IHAs) present with hypoxic bradycardia due to a primary respiratory aetiology (e.g. pulmonary embolism, excessive sedation). In hospital patients, regular review of **resuscitation status** avoids inappropriate CPR. Good medical management (e.g. avoiding hypoxaemia) may **prevent CPA**, which is always more effective than CPR.

Basic life support

Basic life support (BLS) maintains oxygen supply to vital organs (e.g. brain) until medical treatment (see below) restores spontaneous ventilation and circulation. First assess the arrest scene to exclude and minimize potential danger, call for help and establish whether the patient is responsive (i.e. shout 'Are you all right?' and shake the shoulders avoiding excessive head movement). In unresponsive patients summon medical assistance (i.e. hospital cardiac arrest team). Then assess:

1 *Airway.* Clear the oropharynx of foreign bodies and vomitus (i.e turn head to the side; sweep finger around mouth). Maintain **airway patency** with head tilt, chin lift and jaw thrust (Chapter 7). This prevents the tongue obstructing the pharynx.

2 *Breathing.* 'Look, listen and feel' (i.e. place your cheek and ear over the patient's nose and mouth whilst watching chest wall movement).

3 *Circulation.* Whilst assessing breathing feel for the carotid pulse for 10 s.

Figure (a) summarizes further management according to findings. Responsive but obtunded patients are rolled into the recovery position, but avoid exacerbating other injuries.

Cardiopulmonary resuscitation

Absence of breathing necessitates **artificial ventilation**. During OHA '**mouth-to-mouth**' ventilation may be required. Whilst performing 'chin lift', pinch the nose and maintain slight neck extension by gentle pressure on the forehead. Take a deep breath and place your lips around the patient's mouth, creating an airtight seal. Breathe out slowly, observing chest movement. Allow adequate time for deflation between breaths. If the chest does not move adequately, check technique and exclude airway obstruction. During IHA, '**valve bag, mask ventilation**' followed by intubation is more appropriate (Chapters 7, 9). Absence of a pulse requires **external cardiac massage** (ECM). The heel of one hand is placed two fingers above the xiphoid sternum. The other hand is placed on the first and the fingers interlocked (Fig. b(i)). With the shoulders directly over the hands and the elbows extended, the weight of the body (i.e. not elbow flexion–extension) produces chest compressions (Fig. b(ii)). The sternum is depressed 4–5 cm for 15 compressions at a rate of ~100/min. Then ventilate again for 2 breaths before a further 15 compressions (Fig. b(iii)). The compression : ventilation ratio remains unchanged with two people. An initial precordial thump generates a small electrical shock, but should only be employed for monitored or witnessed arrests.

Advanced life support

Advanced life support (ALS) aims to restore spontaneous ventilation and circulation (Fig. c). CPA is due to:

1 *VF/pulseless VT* in ~80% of cases. This has the best prognosis.

2 *Asystole* in ~15% of cases. The prognosis is poor.

3 *Electromechanical dissociation* (EMD) or *pulseless electrical activity* (PEA) in <5%. This describes an ECG rhythm with no associated cardiac output. When it is cardiac in origin the prognosis is poor but treatable causes (e.g. dynamic hyperinflation, pulmonary embolism) must be excluded.

The CPR team

The CPR team requires ~4 people to undertake the primary ALS activities of: (i) airways management and ventilation; (ii) cardioversion; (iii) circulatory support; (iv) establishing intravenous access and blood gas sampling; (v) preparation and administration of drugs; (vi) special procedures (e.g. chest tube, pacemaker insertion); and (vii) timing and documentation. A team leader supervises, coordinates and prioritizes activity.

ALS management priorities

Connection to a **monitor** and immediate **defibrillation** (Fig. c) are always the **main priorities** if VF is present. BLS continues during ALS but must not delay defibrillation. Following **intubation**, ventilate with 100% oxygen. Hyperventilation corrects acidosis. ECM should be continuous after intubation. Establish **venous access** through a central vein if possible. Alternatively, use a large peripheral vein. If venous access is impossible, some drugs (e.g. adrenaline (epinephrine), lidocaine, atropine) can be administered through the endotracheal tube using double doses.

• **Arrhythmias** are treated as in Chapter 19.

• **Specific therapies** include blood transfusion following haemorrhage (e.g. gastrointestinal bleeding), fluid replacement for suspected hypovolaemia (avoid dextrose infusions) and correction of electrolyte imbalance. Treat tension pneumothorax and cardiac tamponade immediately (Chapters 22, 28). Pulmonary emboli (Chapter 27) may fragment and move peripherally during ECM, reducing haemodynamic effects.

• **Post-resuscitation care.** Review an ECG to exclude myocardial ischaemia and monitor cardiac rhythm for arrhythmias. Assess vital functions including urine output. Arrange a CXR to check line and endotracheal tube positions and exclude pneumothorax.

Prognosis

Most successful CPR requires only 2–3 min. Establishing a patent airway and early defibrillation are the only actions necessary in many CPA survivors. After ~5–6 min success rates are <5% (Fig. d) with the notable exceptions of hypothermia and near-drowning when survival may follow several hours of CPR. **Poor prognostic factors** include: (i) initial rhythms of asystole or bradycardia (i.e. non-VF); (ii) >5 min to onset of BLS or delayed defibrillation; (iii) poor prearrest health or underlying organ dysfunction; (iv) arrest location (i.e. OHA); (v) peri-arrest hyperglycaemia; (vi) antecedent sepsis, renal failure or pneumonia. Interestingly, age alone does not predict outcome.

CPR is highly effective when applied promptly during IHA for electrical instability (i.e. VF in ICU). Nevertheless, **<10% of all CPR cases** and **<3% of OHA victims** survive to hospital discharge without neurological impairment. Although circulatory function is restored in ~40–50% of CPA victims, only ~70% of these 'successes' survive to 24 h and only ~50% reawaken. Recovery of consciousness is greatest in the first 24 h and then declines exponentially. Serious, permanent neurological damage affects ~50% of conscious survivors. Immediately after CPR, absence of pupillary and oculomotor responses indicates an adverse outcome. Defective motor responses predict non-functional recovery best after 24 h.

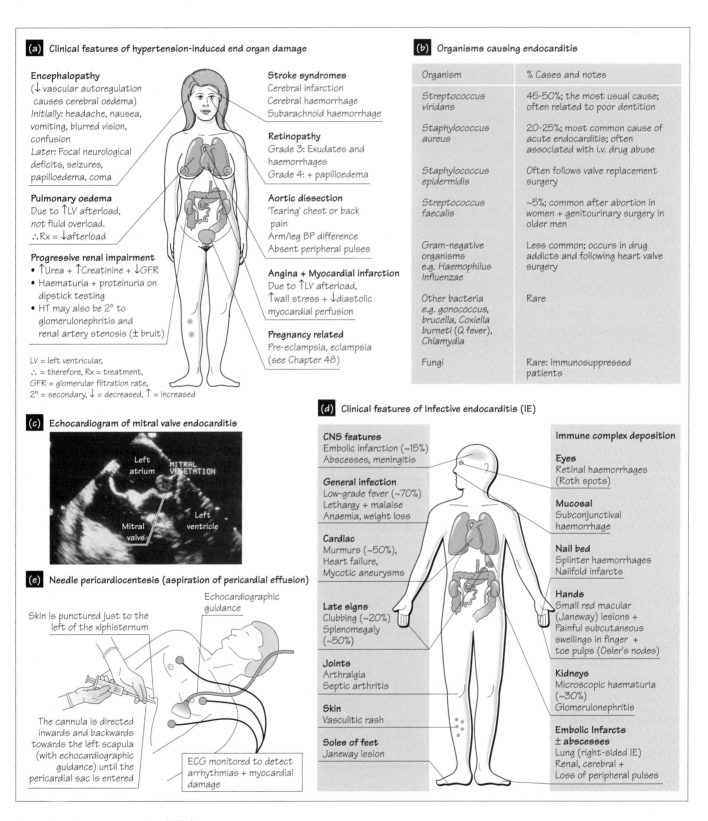

(a) Clinical features of hypertension-induced end organ damage

Encephalopathy
(↓ vascular autoregulation causes cerebral oedema)
Initially: headache, nausea, vomiting, blurred vision, confusion
Later: Focal neurological deficits, seizures, papilloedema, coma

Pulmonary oedema
Due to ↑LV afterload, not fluid overload.
∴ Rx = ↓afterload

Progressive renal impairment
• ↑Urea + ↑Creatinine + ↓GFR
• Haematuria + proteinuria on dipstick testing
• HT may also be 2° to glomerulonephritis and renal artery stenosis (± bruit)

LV = left ventricular,
∴ = therefore, Rx = treatment,
GFR = glomerular filtration rate,
2° = secondary, ↓ = decreased, ↑ = increased

Stroke syndromes
Cerebral infarction
Cerebral haemorrhage
Subarachnoid haemorrhage

Retinopathy
Grade 3: Exudates and haemorrhages
Grade 4: + papilloedema

Aortic dissection
'Tearing' chest or back pain
Arm/leg BP difference
Absent peripheral pulses

Angina + Myocardial infarction
Due to ↑LV afterload,
↑wall stress + ↓diastolic myocardial perfusion

Pregnancy related
Pre-eclampsia, eclampsia
(see Chapter 48)

(b) Organisms causing endocarditis

Organism	% Cases and notes
Streptococcus viridans	45-50%; the most usual cause; often related to poor dentition
Staphylococcus aureus	20-25%; most common cause of acute endocarditis; often associated with i.v. drug abuse
Staphylococcus epidermidis	Often follows valve replacement surgery
Streptococcus faecalis	~5%; common after abortion in women + genitourinary surgery in older men
Gram-negative organisms e.g. *Haemophilus influenzae*	Less common; occurs in drug addicts and following heart valve surgery
Other bacteria e.g. gonococcus, brucella, *Coxiella burneti* (Q fever), Chlamydia	Rare
Fungi	Rare: Immunosuppressed patients

(c) Echocardiogram of mitral valve endocarditis

Left atrium
MITRAL VEGETATION
Mitral valve
Left ventricle

(e) Needle pericardiocentesis (aspiration of pericardial effusion)

Echocardiographic guidance

Skin is punctured just to the left of the xiphisternum

The cannula is directed inwards and backwards towards the left scapula (with echocardiographic guidance) until the pericardial sac is entered

ECG monitored to detect arrhythmias + myocardial damage

(d) Clinical features of Infective endocarditis (IE)

CNS features
Embolic infarction (~15%)
Abscesses, meningitis

General infection
Low-grade fever (~70%)
Lethargy + malaise
Anaemia, weight loss

Cardiac
Murmurs (~50%),
Heart failure,
Mycotic aneurysms

Late signs
Clubbing (~20%)
Splenomegaly (~50%)

Joints
Arthralgia
Septic arthritis

Skin
Vasculitic rash

Soles of feet
Janeway lesion

Immune complex deposition

Eyes
Retinal haemorrhages (Roth spots)

Mucosal
Subconjunctival haemorrhage

Nail bed
Splinter haemorrhages
Nailfold infarcts

Hands
Small red macular (Janeway) lesions +
Painful subcutaneous swellings in finger +
toe pulps (Osler's nodes)

Kidneys
Microscopic haematuria (~30%)
Glomerulonephritis

Embolic Infarcts ± abscesses
Lung (right-sided IE)
Renal, cerebral +
Loss of peripheral pulses

Hypertensive emergencies (HEs)

Definition. Severe hypertension (HT) is a systolic BP >220 mmHg or a diastolic BP >120 mmHg. **Previous definitions** include '**malig-** **nant**' HT with severe HT advanced retinopathy ± organ damage and '**accelerated**' HT with diastolic BP > 140 mmHg, but less retinopathy and organ damage. The best approach is to classify

HE by the presence or absence of **life-threatening organ damage** (LTOD), which determines the urgency for treatment. When LTOD is present (e.g. aortic dissection), BP is reduced to safe levels (diastolic BP ~100 mmHg) within relatively short periods. However, rapid BP reductions can cause strokes, accelerated renal failure and myocardial ischaemia. Consequently, gradual BP reduction is preferable in the absence of LTOD.

Pathophysiology. Most organ damage is due to arteriolar necrotizing vasculitis with platelet and fibrin deposition and loss of vascular autoregulation. **Aetiology:** Inadequate or discontinued therapy for benign essential HT is the commonest cause of HE. However, young (<30 years) or black patients may have secondary causes for severe HT, including renovascular disease, endocrine syndromes (Chapter 33), phaeochromocytoma or drug-induced (e.g. cocaine) catecholamine release. Pregnancy-related HT is discussed in Chapter 48.

Clinical features of HT-induced organ damage are illustrated in Fig. (a). **Prognosis:** The 1-year mortality is >90% if severe HT with LTOD is untreated.

Management. Severe HT with LTOD is a medical emergency requiring admission for close **monitoring.** *Rarely*, immediate BP reduction is required (e.g. dissecting aneurysm) using potent, titratable, short-acting intravenous vasodilator infusions. In these circumstances, invasive arterial BP monitoring is mandatory.

Intravenous therapies include: (i) *Sodium nitroprusside*, an effective and rapidly reversible arteriovenous dilator. Always administer by infusion pump to avoid hypotensive episodes. Prolonged use can cause cyanide poisoning. (ii) *Glyceryl trinitrate*, an arteriovenous dilator, is particularly effective when myocardial ischaemia and pulmonary oedema coexist. (iii) *Labetalol*, an α + β-blocker, is valuable for hypertensive encephalopathy but may exacerbate asthma, heart failure and heart block.

Rarely used agents (e.g. hydralazine, diazoxide) are difficult to titrate as they have prolonged actions. ACE inhibitors can cause severe hypotension and should not be used in this situation.

Severe HT in the absence of LTOD (e.g. severe HT with gradual renal failure) rarely presents the same therapeutic crisis. Whenever possible, **oral** antihypertensive regimes should be used to lower diastolic BP to ~100 mmHg over ~24–48 h. Sublingual **nifedipine** is popular as it has a rapid onset of action, short half-life and is titratable. Oral β-blockers, ACE inhibitors and calcium antagonists are introduced as normal.

Infective endocarditis

Infection of heart valves or endocardium is usually **subacute** and causes a chronic illness when due to non-virulent organisms (e.g. *Streptococcus viridans*). However, it can be **acute** with a fulminant course when due to virulent organisms (e.g. *Staphylococcus*). Figure (b) lists organisms causing infective endocarditis.

Aetiology and pathogenesis. It is most common in elderly people with degenerative aortic and mitral valve disease but also affects patients with prosthetic valves, rheumatic or congenital heart disease. Abnormal valves are particularly susceptible to infection following dental or surgical procedures. Normal valves are occasionally infected by virulent organisms (e.g. *Staphylococcus*).

Clinical features are shown in Fig. (d). Infective endocarditis should be suspected in patients with fever, heart murmurs, anaemia, flu-like symptoms or weight loss. **Systemic embolization** causes splenic, lung, renal and cerebral infarcts (± abscesses). **Immune complex deposition** produces nail bed splinter haemorrhages, retinal haemorrhage (Roth spots), mucosal haemorrhage (e.g. subconjunctival) and painful nodular lesions in finger pulps (Osler's nodes). Microscopic haematuria and splenomegaly are common.

Diagnosis is mainly clinical and confirmed by anaemia, raised ESR or CRP, microscopic haematuria, positive blood cultures (~50–80%) and echocardiography. Transthoracic echocardiography (Fig. c) detects <50% of vegetations. Transoesophageal studies are more sensitive.

Management. Look for and treat underlying infection (e.g. dental abscesses) and send repeated blood cultures. Antibiotic therapy is started with benzylpenicillin and an aminoglycoside and adjusted when the results of blood cultures and minimum inhibitory concentrations are available. Treatment is usually for at least 6 weeks.

Surgery is usually required to replace infected prosthetic valves and native valves when infection or heart failure occurs.

Prognosis. In developed countries, the high mortality (~15%) is due to prosthetic valve infection. **Prophylactic antibiotics** are given to patients with valvular heart disease before dental or potentially septic procedures (e.g. cystoscopy).

Pericardial emergencies

- **Acute pericarditis** is due to infection (most commonly viral), MI, uraemia, connective tissue diseases, trauma, TB or neoplasia. An immunologically mediated febrile pleuropericarditis (Dressler's syndrome) can occur 2–6 weeks after MI (~2%).

Clinical features include severe, positional (i.e. better sitting forward), retrosternal chest pain and pericardial rub on auscultation.

Investigation. ECG shows concave ST segment elevation in all leads. Cardiac enzymes may be elevated with myocarditis.

Management. Bed rest and anti-inflammatory medication (e.g. aspirin). Corticosteroids are required occasionally (e.g. Dressler's syndrome).

- **Pericardial effusion** is due to infection (e.g. TB), uraemia, MI (e.g. Dressler's syndrome), aortic dissection, myxoedema, neoplasia and radiotherapy.

Clinical features are due to cardiac tamponade which occurs when pericardial fluid impairs ventricular filling, reducing CO. Breathlessness and pericarditis often precede acute cardiovascular collapse. Examination may reveal venous congestion which increases on inspiration (Kussmaul's sign), hypotension with a paradoxical pulse (i.e. BP falls >15 mmHg during inspiration) and distant heart sounds.

Investigation. ECG (reduced voltage), CXR (globular cardiomegaly) and echocardiography (pericardial fluid and tamponade-induced right ventricular diastolic collapse) are diagnostic.

Management. Echocardiography-directed, pericardial drainage is required for tamponade (Fig. e).

- **Constrictive pericarditis.** Progressive fibrotic constriction may follow pericarditis, causing pericardial tamponade. Surgical removal of the pericardium may be necessary.

Other cardiac emergencies

Acute valve lesions, type A ascending aorta dissections, trauma (Chapter 46), myocarditis and congenital heart disease may also present as cardiac emergencies.

23 Pneumonia

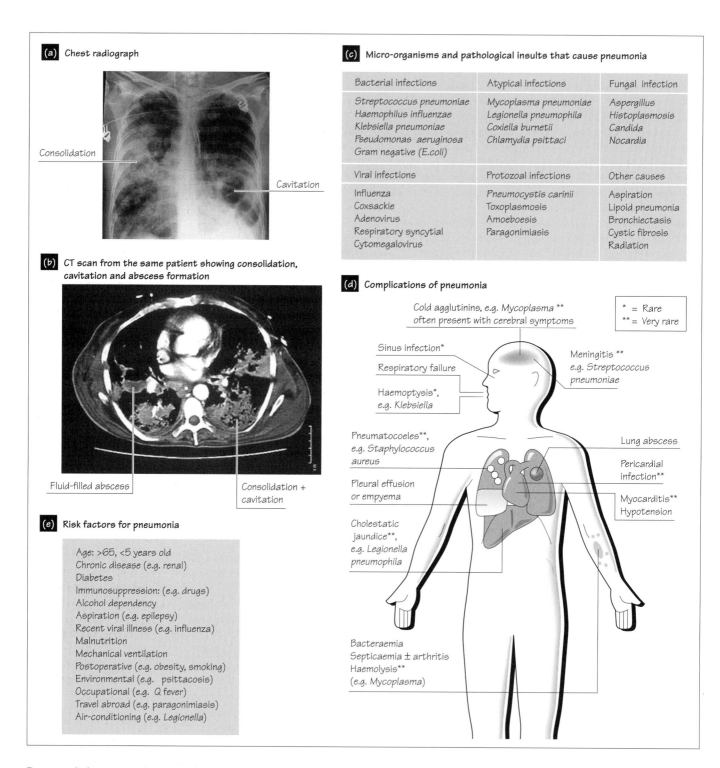

(a) Chest radiograph

Consolidation

Cavitation

(b) CT scan from the same patient showing consolidation, cavitation and abscess formation

Fluid-filled abscess

Consolidation + cavitation

(c) Micro-organisms and pathological insults that cause pneumonia

Bacterial infections	Atypical infections	Fungal infection
Streptococcus pneumoniae	Mycoplasma pneumoniae	Aspergillus
Haemophilus influenzae	Legionella pneumophila	Histoplasmosis
Klebsiella pneumoniae	Coxiella burnetii	Candida
Pseudomonas aeruginosa	Chlamydia psittaci	Nocardia
Gram negative (E.coli)		
Viral infections	**Protozoal infections**	**Other causes**
Influenza	Pneumocystis carinii	Aspiration
Coxsackie	Toxoplasmosis	Lipoid pneumonia
Adenovirus	Amoeboesis	Bronchiectasis
Respiratory syncytial	Paragonimiasis	Cystic fibrosis
Cytomegalovirus		Radiation

(d) Complications of pneumonia

Cold agglutinins, e.g. Mycoplasma ** often present with cerebral symptoms

* = Rare
** = Very rare

Sinus infection*

Respiratory failure

Meningitis **
e.g. Streptococcus pneumoniae

Haemoptysis*,
e.g. Klebsiella

Pneumatocoeles**,
e.g. Staphylococcus aureus

Lung abscess

Pericardial infection**

Pleural effusion or empyema

Myocarditis**
Hypotension

Cholestatic jaundice**,
e.g. Legionella pneumophila

Bacteraemia
Septicaemia ± arthritis
Haemolysis**
(e.g. Mycoplasma)

(e) Risk factors for pneumonia

Age: >65, <5 years old
Chronic disease (e.g. renal)
Diabetes
Immunosuppression: (e.g. drugs)
Alcohol dependency
Aspiration (e.g. epilepsy)
Recent viral illness (e.g. influenza)
Malnutrition
Mechanical ventilation
Postoperative (e.g. obesity, smoking)
Environmental (e.g. psittacosis)
Occupational (e.g. Q fever)
Travel abroad (e.g. paragonimiasis)
Air-conditioning (e.g. Legionella)

Pneumonia is an acute lower respiratory tract (LRT) illness, usually due to infection, associated with fever, focal chest symptoms (± signs) and recent shadowing on CXR (Fig. a). Table (c) lists microorganisms and pathological insults that cause pneumonia.

Classification

In the clinical situation, microbiological classification of pneumonia is not practical as causative organisms may not be identified or diagnosis takes several days. Likewise, radiographic appearance gives little practical information about cause. The following classification is widely accepted.

• **Community-acquired pneumonia (CAP)** describes LRT infections occurring within 48 h of hospital admission or in patients who have not been hospitalized in the previous 14 days. Likely pathogens are *Streptococcus pneumoniae* (60–75%), *Mycoplasma pneumoniae* (5–18%), influenza A (7–8%), *Haemophilus influenzae* (4–5%) and *Legionella* (2–5%). Alcoholic, diabetic or heart failure patients are prone to *Klebsiella*, staphylococci and Gram-negative organisms. Staphylococcal infection may follow influenza, and *H. influenzae* causes many COPD exacerbations.

• **Hospital-acquired (nosocomial) pneumonia (HAP)** describes any LRT infection developing 2 or more days after hospital admission. Likely organisms are Gram-negative bacilli including *Klebsiella*, *Pseudomonas*, *E. coli*, *Proteus* (65–70%) and *Staphylococcus* (10–15%). Oropharyngeal colonization with these organisms occurs in many hospital patients (>50%) and aspiration due to reduced consciousness or difficulty swallowing may cause LRT infection. **Ventilator-associated pneumonia** often follows prolonged (>8 days) mechanical ventilation and is partly due to leakage of nasopharyngeal secretions or gastric contents past the endotracheal tube.

• **Aspiration pneumonia.** *Bacteroides* and other anaerobic infections follow aspiration of gastric contents due to impaired laryngeal competence (e.g. CVA) or reduced consciousness (e.g. drugs).

• **Pneumonia during immunosuppression** (Chapter 43). HIV, chemotherapy and bone marrow transplant patients are susceptible to viral (e.g. CMV), fungal (e.g. *Aspergillus*) and mycobacterial infections, in addition to the normal range of organisms. HIV patients with CD_4 counts <200/mm^3 are at risk of **opportunistic infections** (e.g. *Pneumocystis carinii* pneumonia (PCP)).

• **Recurrent pneumonia** with aerobic and anaerobic organisms occurs in cystic fibrosis and bronchiectasis.

Epidemiology and risk factors

Incidence. In the UK, ~90% of CAP is treated at home but ~60 000 cases (~1/1000 population) are admitted to hospital annually. HAP causes 15% of hospital-acquired infections and is the third commonest cause after wound and urinary tract infections.

Mortality is 5–18% in hospitalized CAP patients and ~20–30% in HAP cases, rising to ~50% in those with bacteraemia.

Risk factors are reported in Fig. (e). **Specific risk factors** are: **occupational** (e.g. brucellosis in abattoir workers, Q fever in sheep workers); **environmental** (e.g. psittacosis with pet birds, tularaemia and erlichiosis from scrubland or forest tick bites); **geographical** (e.g. coccidomycosis in south-west USA); or **localized** (e.g. *Legionella pneumophila* (Legionnaire's disease) outbreaks may involve a specific hotel due to air-conditioner contamination).

Seasonal variation. Pneumonia is more common in winter due to an increased incidence of viral infections (e.g. influenza). Seasonal peaks (e.g. *Mycoplasma* in autumn, *Staphylococcus* in spring) and annual cycles (e.g. 4-yearly *Mycoplasma* epidemics) are recognized.

Diagnosis

The aims are to establish the diagnosis, determine severity, identify complications and assess aetiology to aid in choosing antibacterial therapy. **In critically ill patients**, diagnosis is difficult because fever, leukocytosis and radiographic features (e.g. oedema, effusions, atelectasis, aspiration) may be non-specific and previous antibiotics limit the value of microbiology.

• **Clinical features.** Symptoms may be general (e.g. fever, rigors, myalgia) or chest specific (e.g. dyspnoea, pleurisy, cough, dis-coloured sputum). Signs include cyanosis, tachycardia and tachypnoea, with focal dullness, crepitations, bronchial breathing and pleuritic rub on chest examination. In young or old patients and during atypical pneumonias (e.g. *Mycoplasma*, *Legionella*), non-respiratory features including headache, confusion and diarrhoea may predominate. **Complications** are illustrated in Fig. (d).

• **Severity assessment.** In CAP the following features are associated with increased mortality and indicate the need for careful monitoring on HDU or ICU. **(a) Clinical:** age >60 years, RR > 30/min, diastolic BP (DBP) <60 mmHg, new atrial fibrillation, confusion and multilobar involvement. **(b) Laboratory:** urea >7 mmol/L, albumin <35 g/L, hypoxaemia (Po_2 < 8 kPa), leucopenia (WCC < 4×10^9/L), leucocytosis (>20×10^9/L) and bacteraemia. The risk of death is increased 20-fold if two of RR > 30/min, DBP < 60 mmHg or urea >7 mmol/L are present.

• **Investigation.** No microorganism is isolated in ~33–50% of patients due to previous antibiotic therapy or inadequate specimens. Include: **routine blood tests:** haemolysis and cold agglutinins indicate *Mycoplasma* infection; abnormal liver function tests suggest *Legionella* or *Mycoplasma* infection. **Blood gases** to assess respiratory failure (Chapters 6, 12). **Microbiology:** Blood cultures, sputum and non-directed bronchoalveolar lavage may identify the pathogen and antibiotic sensitivity. **Serology** identifies *Mycoplasma* infection but long processing times limit clinical value. Rapid detection of *Legionella* antigen in urine and pneumococcal antigen in serum, pleural fluid or urine may be useful. **Radiological:** CXR and computed tomography (CT) scans aid diagnosis, indicate severity and detect complications (Fig. a). Radiographic changes lag behind clinical features in atypical pneumonias.

Management

Supportive measures include oxygen to maintain P_aO_2 > 8 kPa (saturation <90%) and intravenous fluids (±inotropes) to ensure haemodynamic stability (Chapters 5, 6).

Ventilatory support. Non-invasive or mechanical ventilation may be required in respiratory failure (Chapters 8, 10).

Physiotherapy and bronchoscopy aid sputum clearance (Ch. 11).

Initial antibiotic therapy represents the 'best guess', according to pneumonia classification and likely organisms, as microbiological results are often not available for >24 h. Therapy is adjusted when results and antibiotic sensitivities are available. The American and British Thoracic Societies (ATS, BTS) have recommended initial treatment protocols.

• **CAP.** In hospitalized patients, antibiotic therapy must cover atypical pneumonias and *S. pneumoniae*. Erythromycin (or another macrolide) alone (ATS) or combined with cefuroxime (BTS) is recommended. Therapy may need to cover staphylococcal infection following influenza and *H. influenzae* in COPD.

• **HAP.** Treat Gram-negative bacilli and staphylococci, using combinations of two or three broad-spectrum antibiotics (e.g. cephalosporins, quinolones, antistaphylococcal drugs).

• **Other pneumonias.** Following aspiration, therapy should also cover anaerobes (e.g. metronidazole). Immunocompromised patients require antifungal, antiviral and broad-spectrum antibiotic regimes. PCP is treated with steroids and high-dose co-trimoxazole. HIV patients may need specific therapy for protozoal infections (Chapter 43).

24 Asthma

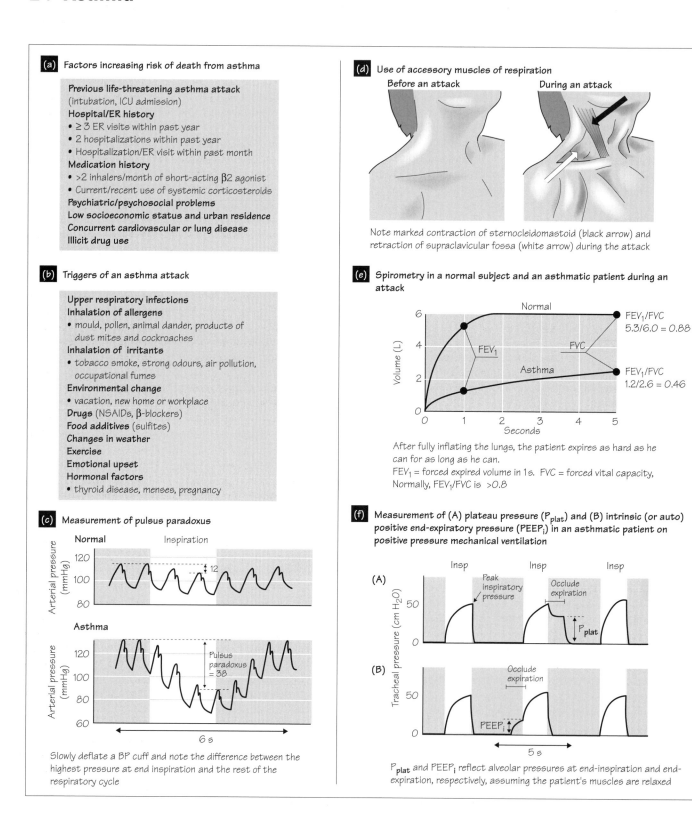

(a) Factors increasing risk of death from asthma

Previous life-threatening asthma attack
(intubation, ICU admission)
Hospital/ER history
• ≥ 3 ER visits within past year
• 2 hospitalizations within past year
• Hospitalization/ER visit within past month
Medication history
• >2 inhalers/month of short-acting β2 agonist
• Current/recent use of systemic corticosteroids
Psychiatric/psychosocial problems
Low socioeconomic status and urban residence
Concurrent cardiovascular or lung disease
Illicit drug use

(b) Triggers of an asthma attack

Upper respiratory infections
Inhalation of allergens
• mould, pollen, animal dander, products of
dust mites and cockroaches
Inhalation of irritants
• tobacco smoke, strong odours, air pollution,
occupational fumes
Environmental change
• vacation, new home or workplace
Drugs (NSAIDs, β-blockers)
Food additives (sulfites)
Changes in weather
Exercise
Emotional upset
Hormonal factors
• thyroid disease, menses, pregnancy

(c) Measurement of pulsus paradoxus

Slowly deflate a BP cuff and note the difference between the
highest pressure at end inspiration and the rest of the
respiratory cycle

(d) Use of accessory muscles of respiration

Note marked contraction of sternocleidomastoid (black arrow) and
retraction of supraclavicular fossa (white arrow) during the attack

(e) Spirometry in a normal subject and an asthmatic patient during an attack

FEV_1/FVC
$5.3/6.0 = 0.88$

FEV_1/FVC
$1.2/2.6 = 0.46$

After fully inflating the lungs, the patient expires as hard as he
can for as long as he can.
FEV_1 = forced expired volume in 1s. FVC = forced vital capacity,
Normally, FEV_1/FVC is >0.8

(f) Measurement of (A) plateau pressure (P_{plat}) and (B) intrinsic (or auto) positive end-expiratory pressure ($PEEP_i$) in an asthmatic patient on positive pressure mechanical ventilation

P_{plat} and $PEEP_i$ reflect alveolar pressures at end-inspiration and end-
expiration, respectively, assuming the patient's muscles are relaxed

Asthma is **reversible obstruction** of inflamed, hyperreactive airways manifested by recurrent episodes of wheezing, coughing and dyspnoea. It affects 5–10% of the population. **Prevalence** is increasing, particularly among black people and children. Although **mortality is low** (2 deaths/year/100 000), it has increased for 20 years and is higher in black people. Factors increasing risk of death are shown in Fig. (a).

Pathogenesis

Airway inflammation is central to pathogenesis. In most cases, inflammation is allergic and may derive from the predominance of type 2 T-helper lymphocytes over type 1 due to genetic–environmental interactions in childhood. Characteristic airway changes include accumulation of inflammatory cells, mediator release, epithelial denudation, oedema and submucosal fibrosis, goblet cell hyperplasia, submucosal gland enlargement, mucous hypersecretion, and hypertrophied hyperresponsive smooth muscle.

Pathophysiology

Acute airway obstruction can be triggered by a variety of factors (Fig. b). During an attack, the patient struggles to keep obstructed airways open by breathing at high lung volumes, using accessory muscles (Fig. d). Work of breathing increases due to high airways resistance, decreased lung compliance and reduced muscle efficiency. Heroic efforts sufficient to increase alveolar ventilation and lower $P_a\text{CO}_2$ despite increasing deadspace fail to maintain airway patency, resulting in hypoxaemia due to regional hypoventilation (i.e. low ventilation/perfusion ratio). Hypoxic vasoconstriction and pulmonary capillary compression cause pulmonary hypertension, increased RV afterload and right heart failure. Increased RV filling pressures may push the interventricular septum into the LV cavity, decreasing LV end-diastolic volume. Marked inspiratory decreases in pleural pressure impair LV emptying. As a result, systolic volume may decrease more than usual during inspiration, causing abnormal reductions ($\geq 15\,\text{mmHg}$) in systolic blood pressure (pulsus paradoxus). If the attack does not abate, respiratory muscles become exhausted, leading to respiratory arrest and death.

Clinical features

Onset of asthma is usually gradual but may be sudden. Episodic wheeze, cough and nocturnal waking with breathlessness are typical. The history may reveal a seasonal pattern, precipitating causes (Fig. b) and risk factors for death (Fig. a). **Physical examination** demonstrates wheeze with prolonged expiration on chest auscultation and signs of hyperinflation (e.g. hyperresonance).

- **Severe asthma** is characterized by a peak expiratory flow rate (PEFR) <50% of predicted, agitation, difficulty completing sentences, respiratory rate >25/min, sweating, accessory muscle use and pulsus paradoxus (Fig. c).
- **Features of life-threatening asthma** that indicate respiratory failure and impending arrest include confusion and drowsiness, silent chest, PEFR <33% of predicted, paradoxical thoracoabdominal excursions (outward abdominal and inward sternal movement during inspiration), bradycardia, hypotension, pulsus paradoxus and hypercapnia (±hypoxaemia).

Investigation

Initially **arterial blood gases** demonstrate hypoxaemia (or normoxia), hypocapnia and alkalosis. A rise in $P_a\text{CO}_2$ suggests impending respiratory muscle fatigue and failure. **Chest radiography** excludes other pathology (e.g. pneumothorax) and assesses endotracheal tube position. **Electrocardiography** may exhibit signs of RV strain. **FEV$_1$** (Fig. e) or **PEFR** are measured to assess severity and monitor therapy.

Management

- **ICU admission** is indicated if severe airways obstruction has worsened following initial therapy, not improved despite treatment for ≥6 h, when respiratory arrest is imminent, or complications (e.g. pneumothorax, arrhythmias) have occurred.
- **Primary pharmacological therapy** is essential in all patients and includes inhaled short-acting **β$_2$-adrenergic agonists** (e.g. albuterol, salbutamol) and **intravenous corticosteroids** which are administered until sustained improvement is achieved. Systemic **β$_2$-adrenergic agonists** (e.g. terbutaline, salbutamol) have no proven advantage over inhaled therapy. Failure to improve within 6–24 h warrants addition of **secondary pharmacological therapy**, although clear evidence for benefit has not been established. Inhaled **ipratropium bromide** reduces airways obstruction caused by cholinergic mechanisms. Intravenous **magnesium sulphate** may improve severe attacks, but should not be used in renal failure or heart block. Use of intravenous **aminophylline** is controversial. It dilates airway smooth muscle and increases respiratory and cardiac muscle contractility through inhibition of phosphodiesterases; however, close monitoring of serum levels and dose adjustments are required to avoid serious toxic effects (e.g. seizures).
- **Respiratory therapy** aims to establish adequate oxygenation and relieve dyspnoea. All patients should receive sufficient **oxygen** by facemask or nasal cannula to correct hypoxaemia (usually ≤50% or 6 L/min, respectively). **Non-invasive positive pressure ventilation** (Chapter 8) may alleviate respiratory muscle fatigue and improve gas exchange. Using tight-fitting face masks, modest levels of positive pressure are administered during expiration (5–10 cmH$_2$O) and inspiration (10–15 cmH$_2$O) to decrease the effort required to initiate and sustain airflow into hyperinflated lungs, where end-expiratory alveolar pressure may exceed atmospheric pressure (intrinsic or auto-PEEP). *Risks* include worsened hyperinflation, agitation, aspiration and facial skin necrosis. Occasionally, removing mucus plugs by **bronchoalveolar lavage** may relieve obstruction.
- **Mechanical ventilation** is required in ventilatory failure, coma or cardiopulmonary arrest (Chapters 9, 10). Deep **sedation** allows **controlled hypoventilation**, a strategy which decreases hyperinflation by increasing expiratory time (Chapter 11). Resulting CO$_2$ retention, due to reduced minute ventilation, is termed 'permissive hypercapnia' and occasionally respiratory acidosis (pH < 7.2) may require correction with sodium bicarbonate. Paralytic agents interact with corticosteroids to cause postparalytic myopathy (Chapter 40) but cannot always be avoided. A volume-controlled mode of ventilation is used in patients making few respiratory efforts, or intermittent mandatory ventilation if respiratory efforts are not reduced by sedation. In both modes, the rate and volume of ventilator breaths should be minimized (usually ≤10/min and ≤6 mL/kg, respectively). Inspiratory flow should be maximized (≥100 L/min) but the resulting increase in peak inspiratory pressure (usually ≥50 cmH$_2$O) should not cause this strategy to be abandoned. Better indicators of lung volume are the plateau pressure (P_{plat}) and the level of intrinsic or auto-PEEP (PEEP$_i$), measured as shown in Fig. (f) to estimate alveolar pressure at end-inspiration and end-expiration, respectively. Safe levels are unknown, but $P_{\text{plat}} < 30$ and PEEP$_i < 10$ cmH$_2$O are likely to reduce risks. Intubated patients who deteriorate may respond to a trial of **general anaesthesia with halothane or isoflurane**.

25 Chronic obstructive pulmonary disease

(a) Risk factors for COPD

Smoking
Age >50 years old; prevalence ~5-10%
Male gender
Childhood chest infections
Airways hyperreactivity
• asthma/atopy
Low socioeconomic status
α_1-Antitrypsin deficiency
Heavy metal exposure
• cadmium
Atmospheric pollution

(b) Pathophysiology of chronic bronchitis and emphysema

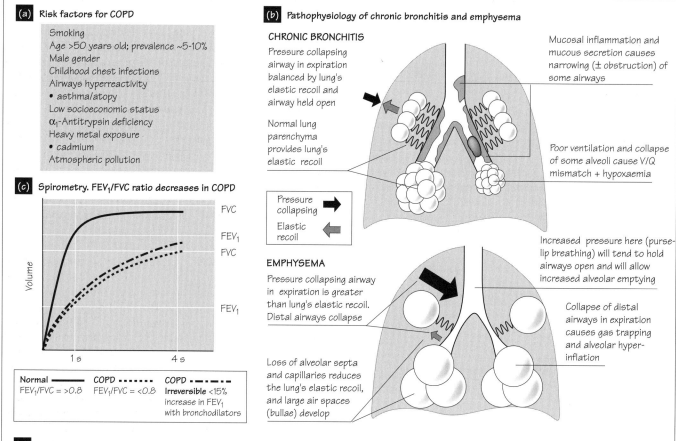

CHRONIC BRONCHITIS

Pressure collapsing airway in expiration balanced by lung's elastic recoil and airway held open

Normal lung parenchyma provides lung's elastic recoil

Mucosal inflammation and mucous secretion causes narrowing (± obstruction) of some airways

Poor ventilation and collapse of some alveoli cause V/Q mismatch + hypoxaemia

Pressure collapsing ➡
Elastic recoil ➡

EMPHYSEMA

Pressure collapsing airway in expiration is greater than lung's elastic recoil. Distal airways collapse

Loss of alveolar septa and capillaries reduces the lung's elastic recoil, and large air spaces (bullae) develop

Increased pressure here (purse-lip breathing) will tend to hold airways open and will allow increased alveolar emptying

Collapse of distal airways in expiration causes gas trapping and alveolar hyper-inflation

(c) Spirometry. FEV$_1$/FVC ratio decreases in COPD

Volume

FVC
FEV$_1$
FVC

FEV$_1$

1 s   4 s

Normal ——	COPD •••••••	COPD —•—•—
FEV$_1$/FVC = >0.8	FEV$_1$/FVC = <0.8	**Irreversible** <15% increase in FEV$_1$ with bronchodilators

(d) Mechanical ventilation in COPD requires an adequate inspiratory time to ensure alveolar inflation (i); increased expiratory time to prevent gas trapping (ii); ± ventilator (extrinsic) PEEP to balance auto-PEEP and reduce gas trapping and work of breathing (iii)

(i) Adequate inspiratory time
A short inspiratory time: Results in incomplete inflation of alveoli with narrowed airways causing V/Q mismatching and hypoxaemia

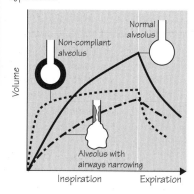

Normal alveolus
Non-compliant alveolus
Volume
Alveolus with airways narrowing
Inspiration   Expiration

Time constant (TC) determines alveolar filling
Time constant = compliance x resistance
• Non-compliant alveoli have short TC
• Alveoli with narrowed airways have long TC

(ii) Increased expiratory time
A long expiratory time is required to prevent gas trapping because the rate of alveolar deflation is decreased due to:
1. Airways obstruction: which slows expiration. A short expiratory time causes incomplete alveolar emptying (gas trapping)

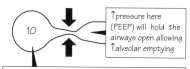

10   Reduced airflow

2. Distal airways collapse: initially reduces airflow and then causes gas trapping (Fig c)

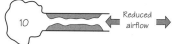

10

↑pressure here (PEEP) will hold the airways open allowing ↑alveolar emptying

The pressure of the trapped gas (intrinsic (or auto) PEEP) can be measured at end expiration by occluding the expiratory limb of the ventilator

A reduction in breath rate (8-10/min) increases both inspiratory and expiratory times

(iii) Reduced work of breathing (WoB)
Hyperinflation increases WoB which can be reduced by bronchodilation, ↑expiratory time (i.e. ↓ breath rate) and ventilator (extrinsic) PEEP matched to auto-PEEP

No PEEP added

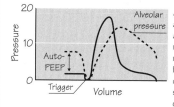

20
Pressure
10
0

Auto-PEEP ↓
Trigger   Volume
Alveolar pressure

Auto-PEEP represents an end-expiratory alveolar pressure that must be overcome by respiratory effort before the ventilator can be triggered or spontaneous breathing can begin

5 cm H$_2$O PEEP added

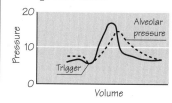

20
Pressure
10
0

Trigger
Volume
Alveolar pressure

PEEP similar to the auto-PEEP added downstream from the site of flow limitation does not significantly slow expiratory airflow but reduces the inspiratory work of breathing

Chronic obstructive pulmonary disease (COPD) encompasses emphysema and chronic bronchitis. It is characterized by irreversible, expiratory airflow obstruction and increased work of breathing. Typically, smoking and other risk factors (Fig. a) accelerate the normal age-related decline in expiratory airflow and cause chronic respiratory symptoms, disability and respiratory failure punctuated by intermittent acute exacerbations.

Pathophysiology

Although emphysema and chronic bronchitis often coexist they are different processes. **Emphysema** destroys **alveolar septa and capillaries** and may be due to inadequate antiprotease defences. Smoking causes *centrilobular* emphysema with mainly upper lobe involvement, whereas α_1-antitrypsin deficiency causes *panacinar* emphysema which affects the lower lobes. Lung tissue loss results in bullae, reduced elastic recoil and impaired diffusion capacity. Airways obstruction is caused by distal airways collapse during expiration due to loss of 'elastic' radial traction from normal lung (Fig. b). Resulting hyperinflation enhances expiratory airflow but inspiratory muscles work at a mechanical disadvantage. **Chronic bronchitic** airways obstruction is due to **chronic mucosal inflammation**, mucous gland hypertrophy with **hypersecretion** and **bronchospasm** (Fig. b). Lung parenchyma is unaffected.

Diagnosis

Spirometry (Fig. c) demonstrates airflow obstruction (**FEV_1:FVC ratio <0.7**) which is largely irreversible with bronchodilator or steroid therapy (i.e. <15% increase in FEV_1). In **emphysema** resting blood gases are usually normal because alveolar septa and capillaries are destroyed in equal proportion. Exercise desaturation and increased minute ventilation are due to reduced diffusion capacity. Lung function tests confirm impaired diffusion ($D_L$co, Kco) and increased lung volumes (TLC, FRC, residual volume). CXR reveals hyperinflation (e.g. flat diaphragms), narrow mediastinum, bullae and reduced vascular markings. In **bronchitis** diffusion capacity and lung volumes are normal but V/Q mismatching may cause hypoxaemia. CXR shows increased vascular markings but normal lung volumes.

Clinical features

The concept of emphysematous **'pink puffers'** and bronchitic **'blue bloaters'** is unreliable as most patients have elements of both. **Emphysematous patients** tend to be **breathless** and **tachypnoeic**, with signs of hyperinflation and malnutrition including *barrel chest*, *purse-lipped breathing* and *accessory muscle use*. Chest auscultation reveals *distant breath sounds* and *prolonged expiratory wheeze*. **Chronic bronchitis** is clinically defined as daily morning cough and mucus production for 3 months over 2 successive years. These patients are less breathless despite potential **hypoxaemia**. Reduced respiratory drive leads to **CO_2 retention** with bounding pulse, vasodilation, confusion, headache, flapping tremor and papilloedema. Hypoxaemia-induced renal fluid retention and right heart failure cause **cor pulmonale** (i.e hepatomegaly, ankle oedema, raised CVP). **Pulmonary hypertension** is a late feature due to hypoxic pulmonary vasoconstriction and extensive capillary loss.

Management

No specific therapy reverses COPD but disease progression can be reduced and symptoms minimized by **smoking cessation**. **Pharmacological therapy:** Inhaled β-agonists (e.g. salbutamol) and anticholinergics (e.g. tiotropium bromide) improve symptoms and lung function. Theophyllines improve exercise tolerance and blood gases but with negligible effects on spirometry. Oral corticosteroids benefit <25% of patients but side-effects limit routine use. Inhaled corticosteroids may be considered in severe disease ($FEV_1 < 1$ L). Mucolytics occasionally help. **Pulmonary rehabilitation** strengthens respiratory muscles, increases exercise tolerance, improves quality of life and reduces hospitalizations without an effect on lung function. **Home oxygen therapy** used for >15 h/day improves survival in hypoxaemic patients. **Prophylaxis:** Pneumococcal and influenza vaccination reduce exacerbations. **Surgery:** Lung volume reduction or transplantation may be indicated in advanced COPD but long-term efficacy is not established. **Prognosis:** Yearly mortality is ~25% when FEV_1 is <0.8 L. This is increased by coexisting cor pulmonale, hypercapnia and weight loss.

Acute exacerbations

The cause is often unknown but infection, pulmonary embolism, IHD, arrhythmias, medications and metabolic disturbances can precipitate exacerbations.

General measures. Fluid management is difficult, especially in cor pulmonale, and requires careful monitoring. Electrolyte correction (e.g. hypokalaemia) and nutrition improve respiratory muscle strength. Thromboembolic prophylaxis is essential. **Oxygen therapy (OT)** relieves life-threatening hypoxia. The small $P_a$co$_2$ increase that occurs in most cases is of no consequence. In a few patients with reduced hypoxic respiratory drive ($\pm$ hypercapnia) OT precipitates hypoventilation and further CO_2 retention. However, on the steep part of the oxyhaemoglobin dissociation curve small P_ao$_2$ increases do not cause much CO_2 retention but significantly increase arterial oxygen content. Monitor the response to OT with blood gases to achieve a P_ao$_2 > 8$ kPa without a substantial rise in $P_a$co$_2$ (Chapters 6, 12). **Pharmacological therapy:** High-dose, aerosolized β-agonists and anticholinergic bronchodilators relieve symptoms and improve gas exchange. Short courses of oral corticosteroids also improve lung function and hasten recovery. Antibiotic therapy is directed at likely organisms (e.g. *H. influenzae*, *S. pneumoniae*) and adjusted according to microbiological results. **Respiratory therapy** increases secretion clearance (Chapter 11). Timely NIV may successfully reverse early respiratory failure. Indications for use are discussed in Chapters 6 and 8. **Mechanical ventilation (MV;** Fig. d) may be life-saving but is often associated with prolonged weaning (Chapter 11) and complications (e.g. pneumothorax). In end-stage COPD it may be appropriate to limit ventilatory support to NIV.

Problems due to MV include dynamic hyperinflation (auto-PEEP) with increased work of breathing, raised intrathoracic pressure and patient–ventilator dysynchrony. Hyperinflation is reduced by bronchodilation, increased expiratory time, decreased minute ventilation and setting ventilator PEEP at a similar level to auto-PEEP (Fig. d). Avoid overventilating patients with CO_2 retention as this causes metabolic alkalosis.

26 Acute respiratory distress syndrome (ARDS)

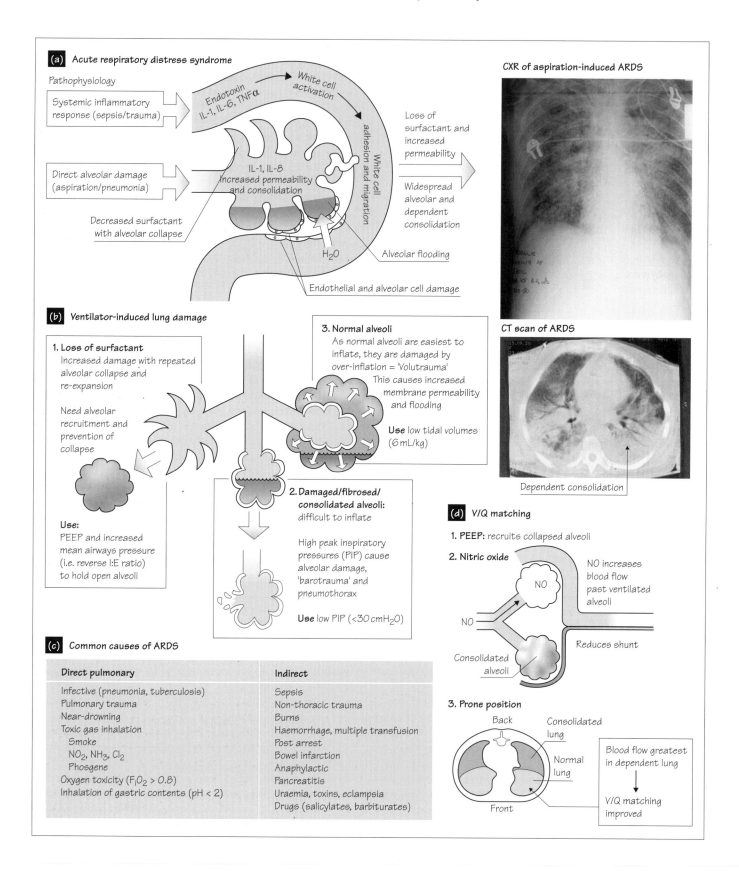

(a) Acute respiratory distress syndrome

Pathophysiology

Systemic inflammatory response (sepsis/trauma) → Endotoxin IL-1, IL-6, TNFα → White cell activation

Direct alveolar damage (aspiration/pneumonia) → IL-1, IL-8 Increased permeability and consolidation

White cell adhesion and migration

Loss of surfactant and increased permeability

Widespread alveolar and dependent consolidation

Decreased surfactant with alveolar collapse

H_2O

Alveolar flooding

Endothelial and alveolar cell damage

CXR of aspiration-induced ARDS

CT scan of ARDS

Dependent consolidation

(b) Ventilator-induced lung damage

1. Loss of surfactant
Increased damage with repeated alveolar collapse and re-expansion

Need alveolar recruitment and prevention of collapse

Use:
PEEP and increased mean airways pressure (i.e. reverse I:E ratio) to hold open alveoli

3. Normal alveoli
As normal alveoli are easiest to inflate, they are damaged by over-inflation = 'Volutrauma'
This causes increased membrane permeability and flooding
Use low tidal volumes (6 mL/kg)

2. Damaged/fibrosed/consolidated alveoli: difficult to inflate

High peak inspiratory pressures (PIP) cause alveolar damage, 'barotrauma' and pneumothorax

Use low PIP (<30 cmH₂O)

(d) V/Q matching

1. **PEEP:** recruits collapsed alveoli
2. **Nitric oxide**

NO

NO

Consolidated alveoli

NO increases blood flow past ventilated alveoli

Reduces shunt

3. **Prone position**

Back

Consolidated lung

Normal lung

Front

Blood flow greatest in dependent lung

↓

V/Q matching improved

(c) Common causes of ARDS

Direct pulmonary	Indirect
Infective (pneumonia, tuberculosis)	Sepsis
Pulmonary trauma	Non-thoracic trauma
Near-drowning	Burns
Toxic gas inhalation	Haemorrhage, multiple transfusion
Smoke	Post arrest
NO_2, NH_3, Cl_2	Bowel infarction
Phosgene	Anaphylactic
Oxygen toxicity ($F_iO_2 > 0.8$)	Pancreatitis
Inhalation of gastric contents (pH < 2)	Uraemia, toxins, eclampsia
	Drugs (salicylates, barbiturates)

ARDS is most simply defined as 'leaky lung syndrome' or 'low pressure (i.e. non-cardiogenic) pulmonary oedema'. It describes acute inflammatory lung injury, often in previously healthy lungs, mediated by a uniform pulmonary pathological process (Fig. a) in response to a variety of direct (i.e. inhaled) or indirect (i.e. blood-borne) insults (Table c). During the **acute inflammatory phase** of ARDS (Fig. a), cytokine-activated neutrophils and monocytes adhere to alveolar epithelium or pulmonary endothelium, releasing inflammatory mediators and proteolytic enzymes. These damage the integrity of the alveolar–capillary membrane, increase permeability and cause alveolar oedema. Reduced surfactant production causes alveolar collapse and hyaline membrane formation. Progressive hypoxaemia and respiratory failure result from loss of functioning alveoli and V/Q mismatch. The later **healing, fibroproliferative phase** causes progressive pulmonary fibrosis and associated pulmonary hypertension.

Diagnosis

The internationally agreed criteria for the diagnosis of ARDS are:
- **severe hypoxaemia** ($P_aO_2/F_iO_2 < 200$ regardless of PEEP); for example, if P_aO_2 is 80 mmHg on 80% inspired oxygen, $P_aO_2/F_iO_2 = 80/0.8 = 100$;
- **bilateral diffuse pulmonary infiltrates on CXR**;
- **normal or only slightly elevated left atrial pressure** (pulmonary artery occlusion pressure <18 mmHg).

Acute lung injury (ALI) is the precursor to ARDS. Apart from a lesser degree of hypoxaemia ($P_aO_2/F_iO_2 < 300$), the criteria for diagnosis are the same.

Epidemiology and prognosis

The incidence of ARDS is ~2–8 cases/100 000 population/year but its precursor ALI is much commoner. Overall **mortality** is high (~50%) but is determined by the precipitating condition (trauma ~35%, sepsis ~55%, aspiration pneumonia ~80%) and increased by age (>60 years) and associated sepsis. The cause of death is multiorgan failure (MOF) and <20% die from hypoxaemia alone.

Clinical features

The **acute inflammatory phase** lasts 3–10 days and results in hypoxaemia and MOF. It presents with progressive breathlessness, tachypnoea, cyanosis, hypoxic confusion and lung crepitations. These features are not diagnostic and are frequently incorrectly interpreted as heart failure. During the **healing, fibroproliferative phase**, lung scarring and pneumothoraces are common. Secondary chest and systemic infections are common in both phases.

Investigation and monitoring

Routine measurements include temperature, respiratory rate, O_2 saturation and urine output. Haemodynamic monitoring, including central venous pressure, cardiac output (CO) and occasionally left atrial pressure (LAP) using a pulmonary artery catheter, ensure appropriate fluid balance and adequate tissue oxygen delivery. Serial blood gases measurement and occasionally capnography are used to monitor gas exchange. Regular microbiological samples (e.g. sputum, bronchial lavage) identify secondary infection early.

Radiology (Fig. a). Serial CXRs detect progression of diffuse bilateral pulmonary infiltrates. Early CT scans often demonstrate dependent consolidation and later scans pneumothoraces, pneumatocoeles and fibrosis.

Management

Management requires identification and treatment of the precipitating cause (e.g. sepsis). In mild disease (e.g. ALI) oxygen therapy, diuretics and physiotherapy maintain gas exchange. If respiratory failure progresses, non-invasive ventilation (Chapter 8) with CPAP improves oxygenation and may avoid the need for MV. However, in severe disease, MV is usually necessary. Due to reduced lung compliance, high PIPs are required to achieve normal tidal volumes (Tv). These high pressures cause lung damage termed 'barotrauma' (e.g. pneumothorax). 'Volutrauma' describes damage to healthy lung or alveoli due to overdistension (Fig. b).
- **Mechanical ventilation** aims to avoid oxygen toxicity (i.e. $F_iO_2 < 80\%$), limit pressure-induced lung damage and volutrauma, optimize alveolar recruitment and oxygenation, and avoid circulatory compromise due to high intrathoracic pressures. A **'protective' lung ventilation strategy** of low Tv (6 mL/kg) and low PIP (<30 cmH$_2$O) prevents lung damage (Chapter 11) whilst high positive end-expiratory pressures (PEEP >10 cmH$_2$O) and long inspiratory to expiratory (I:E) times (i.e. 2:1 instead of the normal 1:2) recruit collapsed alveoli. No ventilatory mode is proven to be superior, although pressure-controlled modes (Chapter 10) are generally favoured. The CO_2 retention, termed 'permissive hypercapnia', resulting from this low tidal volume strategy can usually be tolerated with adequate sedation.
- **Avoid excessive fluid loading** which causes alveolar flooding due to increased alveolar permeability. The aim is to maintain adequate CO and organ perfusion at the lowest possible LAP by using inotropic or vasoactive drugs rather than aggressive fluid filling. In the acute phase, diuretics reduce extravascular lung water and may improve oxygenation.
- **General measures** include good nursing care, physiotherapy, nutrition, sedation and infection control. Metabolic demand is minimized by preventing fever and shivering and controlling agitation with sedatives. No drug therapy including early steroids, anti-inflammatory agents or surfactant has been consistently beneficial in clinical trials of early ARDS. However, 7–10 days after onset, high-dose steroid therapy prevents the development of pulmonary fibrosis.
- **Additional measures** include: **inhaled nitric oxide** which increases perfusion of ventilated alveoli by vasodilating surrounding vessels. This improves V/Q matching and reduces overall shunt fraction (Fig. d). Unfortunately, the initial P_aO_2 improvement is not sustained and there is no survival benefit. **Prone positioning:** As consolidation is usually dependent and blood flow is greatest in the dependent areas, improved V/Q matching can be achieved by turning the patient prone so that non-consolidated, ventilated lung is dependent (Fig. d). **Bronchoscopy** improves ventilation and V/Q matching by removing sputum plugs and secretions. **Extracorporeal membrane oxygenation (ECMO):** Techniques to oxygenate blood or remove CO_2 are effective in children but the benefit in adults has not been established. **Chest drainage:** Air leaks, including pneumothorax and pneumatocoeles, are common during the late fibroproliferative phase and may be difficult to detect on CXR. The importance of CT scanning to localize and drain these has only recently been appreciated (Chapter 28).

27 Deep venous thrombosis and pulmonary embolism

(a) Pulmonary angiograms (A,D) and V/Q scans (B,E = ventilation scans, C,F = perfusion scans) in a normal patient and a patient with a massive right-sided pulmonary embolism. The angiogram (D) shows complete occlusion of the right pulmonary artery. On the V/Q scan there is loss of right lung perfusion (F) but normal ventilation (E)

NORMAL   PULMONARY EMBOLISM

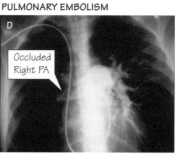
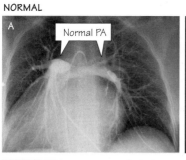

Normal PA

Occluded Right PA

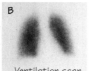
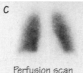
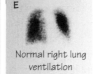
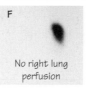

Ventilation scan   Perfusion scan   Normal right lung ventilation   No right lung perfusion

(b) Contrast CT scan showing contrast in the heart and pulmonary arteries (PA). Both the right and left PA show irregular defects consistent with pulmonary emboli

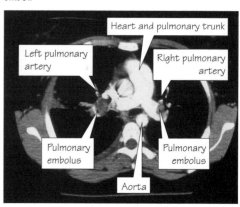

Heart and pulmonary trunk
Left pulmonary artery
Right pulmonary artery
Pulmonary embolus
Pulmonary embolus
Aorta

(c) Risk factors for DVT and PE

Surgery	Hip, knee, gynaecological procedures
Trauma	Spinal trauma
General factors	Age, obesity, smoking, oral contraceptive pill (OCP)
Underlying disease	Malignancy, sepsis, stroke, autoimmune disease
Cardiovascular disease	Low flow states (e.g. cardiac failure, immobility) Vascular injury (e.g. atherosclerosis, catheters)
Inherited disorders (less common)	Deficiencies (e.g. antithrombin III, protein C, protein S) Clotting disorders (e.g. Factor V leiden, antiphospholipid syndrome, dysfibrinogenaemias)

(d) DVT prophylaxis

Risk of DVT	Patient	Regime
Low (<1%)	<40 years old, minor surgery (<1h) Minimal immobility	Early ambulation Compression stockings
Moderate (5-10%)	>40 years old, surgery (>1h), cardiac, medical problems, CVA, hypercoagulability	Low dose heparin (UFH or LMWH)
High (>15%)	Complicated surgery, hip or knee surgery, hip fracture, trauma	Full dose LMWH or warfarin

LMWH = low molecular weight heparin
UFH = unfractionated heparin
CVA = cerebrovascular accident

Virchow's triad of venous stasis, hypercoagulability and vascular injury predispose to deep venous thrombosis (DVT) of which pulmonary embolism (PE) is the most significant complication.

Risk factors for venous thromboembolism (VTE) are listed in Fig. (c). In some settings (e.g. hip or knee replacement surgery) up to 70% of patients who do not receive prophylactic therapy may develop DVT.

Epidemiology. In the USA, ~5 million episodes of DVT occur each year, ~10% embolize and of these ~10% (i.e. 50000) die.

Deep venous thrombosis

Most clinically significant PEs (~90%) arise from DVTs that originate in the calves and propagate above the knees: Clots confined to the calves are of little importance, but the 15–25% that extend into the femoral and iliac veins have ~50% risk of embolizing to the lung. DVT may develop in the axillary and subclavian veins, due to surgery or intravenous catheters, but subsequent emboli are usually smaller with less risk of catastrophic consequences. Soon after formation the intrinsic fibrinolytic cascade begins to organize the thrombus. The risk of embolization is greatest during early clot proliferation and decreases once organized.

Clinical features
Clinical features are non-specific, including pain, heat, swelling and erythema. *Homan's sign*, calf pain on dorsiflexion of the foot, is uncommon. Clinical examination fails to detect at least 50% of DVTs.

Diagnosis
Although venography and iodine-131 fibrinogen scans remain the most sensitive techniques, Doppler ultrasound scanning (USS) is usually the first-line investigation as it is convenient, effective and non-invasive. D-dimers are fibrin degradation products created when fibrin is lysed by plasmin. **D-dimer assays** are sensitive but not specific for DVT as infection, inflammation and malignancy also increase D-dimers. Consequently, a negative D-dimer excludes but cannot confirm VTE.

Prevention
Weight loss, smoking cessation, oral contraceptive pill (OCP) withdrawal and treatment of infection or heart failure should precede elective surgery. Prophylaxis is essential after surgery and in high-risk patients. Therapy depends on the level of risk (Fig. c) and includes pneumatic compression devices, regular leg exercises whilst in bed and early mobilization. Unfractionated heparin (UFH) and low molecular weight heparin (LMWH) reduce the postoperative incidence of DVT by ~50% and of PE by ~65–75%.

Treatment
LMWHs are as effective as heparin therapy at preventing clot extension and PE in established DVT. Subsequent oral anticoagulation with warfarin is required for at least 6 weeks.

Pulmonary embolism
When a thrombus embolizes to the lung, respiratory or circulatory abnormalities occur due to sudden occlusion of pulmonary arteries. Hypoxaemia is mainly due to V/Q mismatch. Pre-existing RV function, rate of onset and degree of pulmonary vascular bed obliteration determine the cardiovascular response. A single large embolus can be catastrophic, whereas multiple small emboli with progressive 'pruning' of pulmonary arteries may be tolerated due to adaptive responses. In general, circulatory collapse occurs with >50% obstruction of the pulmonary arterial bed. Smaller emboli may be fatal when pre-existing lung or heart disease coexists. Pulmonary infarction occurs in <25% of pulmonary emboli.

Clinical presentation
PE presents with pleuritic pain and haemoptysis in ~65%, isolated dyspnoea in ~25% and circulatory collapse in ~10% of cases. Dyspnoea is not present in ~30% of patients with confirmed PE. Other non-specific features include apprehension, tachypnoea, tachycardia, cough, sweating and syncope. With severe PE, signs related to **RV failure** (e.g. hypotension, jugular venous distension) may occur. Most patients have non-specific abnormalities on CXR including atelectasis due to reduced surfactant production in areas of poorly perfused lung.

- The **ECG** may show non-specific ST segment changes and rarely, following a large PE, RV strain with an $S_1Q_3T_3$ pattern, right axis deviation (RAD) or right bundle branch block (RBBB).
- **Arterial blood gas** abnormalities are common, including widened A–a gradient, hypoxaemia and hypocapnia (despite increased dead space).

Diagnosis
Although **pulmonary angiography** remains the diagnostic standard, **V/Q scanning** is usually the initial investigation, as it is less invasive (Fig. a). A negative perfusion scan effectively rules out PE and a 'high probability' scan (multiple segmental perfusion defects with normal ventilation) has a >85% probability of PE. With a high clinical suspicion, a high probability V/Q scan has a positive predictive value >95%. Unfortunately, most V/Q scans are not diagnostic, or indeterminate with a 15–50% likelihood of PE, necessitating further imaging.

- Confirmation of lower limb DVT with **Doppler USS** or **impedance plethysmography** is useful since the presence of thrombosis requires treatment similar to PE. Absence of a DVT combined with a low probability V/Q scan permits withholding of treatment, whereas a negative USS with an intermediate probability V/Q scan (or underlying cardiac or pulmonary disease) necessitates pulmonary CT scanning or angiography.
- **Spiral CT scanning** (Fig. b) has a sensitivity for PE from 70 to 95% (higher for more proximal emboli) and a specificity >90%. It also allows visualization of parenchymal abnormalities and is useful in patients with COPD or extensive CXR abnormalities where V/Q scanning is indeterminate.
- **Magnetic resonance imaging (MRI) scans** are most specific and sensitive but not widely available.
- **Echocardiography** may reveal RV dysfunction, and **transoesophageal echocardiography** detects emboli in the main pulmonary arteries but not in lobar or segmental arteries.

Treatment
Treatment is similar to that for established DVT.
- **Anticoagulation** stops propagation of existing lower limb thrombus and allows organization. Immediate therapy in patients with a high suspicion of PE may prevent further life-threatening emboli. **Heparin (UFH *or* LMWH)** for 5–7 days followed by warfarin for 3–6 months is standard therapy. UFH and warfarin must be monitored as subtherapeutic levels increase the risk of recurrent thromboembolism. LMWH is more bioavailable and does not require monitoring. Patients with inherited or acquired hypercoagulability may require lifelong therapy (Chapter 41).
- If contraindications prevent anticoagulation (e.g. recent surgery, haemorrhagic stroke, CNS metastases, active bleeding) or recurrent PEs occur whilst on therapeutic anticoagulation, an **inferior vena cava filter** may prevent further PE.
- **Thrombolytic therapy** hastens the resolution of perfusion defects and RV dysfunction. In patients without massive PE, increased bleeding complications, including a 0.3–1.5% risk of intracerebral haemorrhage were not associated with improved long-term benefit. Therefore thrombolysis is only recommended in life-threatening PE with compromised haemodynamics.

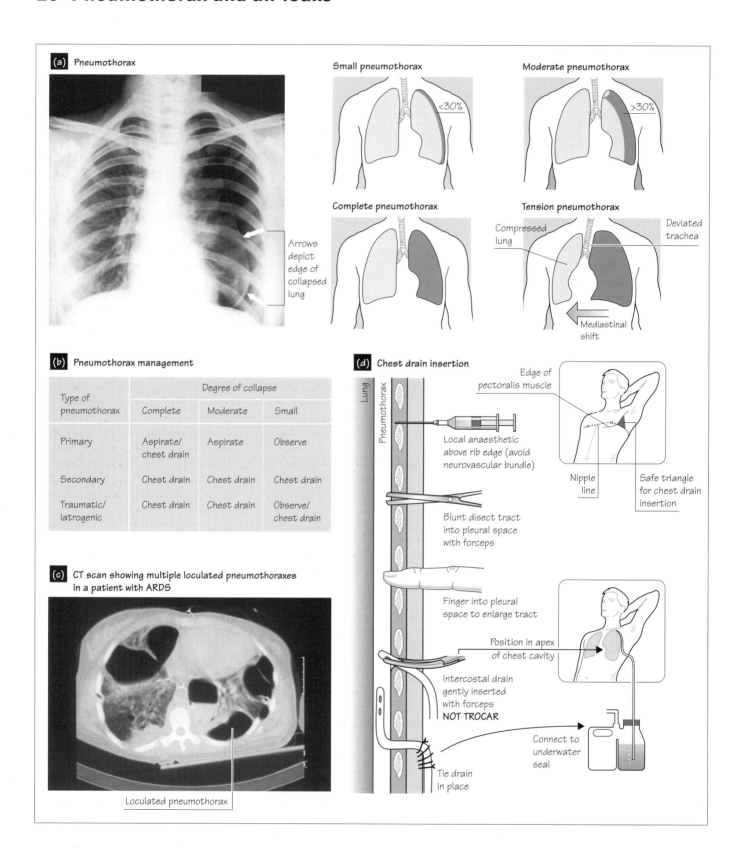

(a) Pneumothorax

Arrows depict edge of collapsed lung

Small pneumothorax
<30%

Moderate pneumothorax
>30%

Complete pneumothorax

Tension pneumothorax

Compressed lung

Deviated trachea

Mediastinal shift

(b) Pneumothorax management

Type of pneumothorax	Degree of collapse		
	Complete	Moderate	Small
Primary	Aspirate/ chest drain	Aspirate	Observe
Secondary	Chest drain	Chest drain	Chest drain
Traumatic/ Iatrogenic	Chest drain	Chest drain	Observe/ chest drain

(c) CT scan showing multiple loculated pneumothoraxes in a patient with ARDS

Loculated pneumothorax

(d) Chest drain insertion

Lung

Pneumothorax

Local anaesthetic above rib edge (avoid neurovascular bundle)

Blunt disect tract into pleural space with forceps

Finger into pleural space to enlarge tract

Intercostal drain gently inserted with forceps **NOT TROCAR**

Tie drain in place

Edge of pectoralis muscle

Nipple line

Safe triangle for chest drain insertion

Position in apex of chest cavity

Connect to underwater seal

Pneumothorax (i.e. a collection of air between the visceral and parietal pleura causing a real rather than potential pleural space) and air leaks are common in critical care units. Recognition and early drainage can be life-saving. Predisposing and precipitating factors include necrotizing lung pathology, ventilator-associated lung injury, chest trauma and cardiothoracic surgery.

Pneumothorax
Classification

1 *Primary spontaneous pneumothorax (PSP)* is caused by rupture of small apical subpleural air cysts ('blebs') but rarely causes significant physiological disturbance. Tall, young (20–40-year-old) men (M:F 5:1) with no underlying lung disease are usually affected. It is the commonest type of pneumothorax (prevalence $8/10^5$/year, rising to $200/10^5$/year in subjects >1.9 m in height). Following a second PSP, recurrence is likely (>60%). Pleurodesis to fuse the visceral and parietal pleura using medical (e.g. pleural insertion of bleomycin or talc) or surgical (e.g. abrasion of the pleural lining) means is recommended.

2 *Secondary pneumothorax (SP)* is associated with respiratory diseases that damage lung architecture, most commonly obstructive (e.g. COPD, asthma), fibrotic or infective (e.g. pneumonia), and occasionally rare or inherited disorders (e.g. Marfan's, cystic fibrosis). The incidence of SP increases with age and the severity of the underlying lung disease. These patients usually require hospital admission as even a small SP in a patient with reduced respiratory reserve may have more serious implications than a large PSP. ICU patients with lung disease are at particular risk of SP due to the high pressures ('barotrauma') and alveolar overdistension ('volutrauma') associated with mechanical ventilation. 'Protective' ventilation strategies using low-pressure, limited-volume ventilation reduce this risk (Chapters 10, 11, 26).

3 *Traumatic (iatrogenic) pneumothorax (TP)* follows blunt (e.g. road traffic accidents) or penetrating (e.g. fractured ribs, stab wounds) chest trauma (Chapter 46). Therapeutic procedures (e.g. line insertion, thoracic surgery) are common causes of iatrogenic pneumothorax.

A **tension pneumothorax** may complicate PSP or SP but is most common during mechanical ventilation and following TP. It occurs when air accumulates in the pleural cavity faster than it can be removed. Increased intrathoracic pressure causes mediastinal shift, compression of functioning lung, inhibition of venous return and shock due to reduced CO. It is a medical emergency and fatal if not rapidly relieved by drainage. Detection is a clinical diagnosis; awaiting CXR confirmation may be life-threatening. Immediate drainage with a 14 G needle in the second intercostal space in the midclavicular line is essential. A characteristic 'hiss' of escaping gas confirms the diagnosis. A chest drain is then inserted.

Clinical assessment

Pneumothorax is graded and treated according to Fig. (a) and Table (b). Sudden breathlessness and/or sharp pleuritic pain suggest a pneumothorax. Most PSPs are small (<30%), and cause few symptoms other than pain. Clinical signs can be surprisingly difficult to detect, but in larger pneumothoraces reduced air entry and hyperresonant percussion over one hemithorax are characteristic and may be associated with tachypnoea and cyanosis. Cardiorespiratory compromise may develop rapidly in a tension pneumothorax or in mechanically ventilated patients and requires immediate drainage. Occasionally other air leaks occur (see below). **Monitoring** reveals tachycardia, hypotension and desaturation. **Blood gases** may demonstrate respiratory failure. **CXR** confirms the diagnosis (Fig. a). **CT scan** may detect localized pneumothoraces following trauma or mechanical ventilation (Fig. c).

Management

Immediate supportive therapy includes supplemental oxygen and analgesia. Treatment depends on cause, size and symptoms.

• A tension pneumothorax must be drained immediately. A small PSP (<30%) is simply observed and spontaneous reabsorption is confirmed on serial outpatient CXR. A PSP >30% may be aspirated through a 16 G needle in the second intercostal space in the midclavicular line using a 50-mL syringe connected to a three-way tap and underwater seal. Following overnight observation, successful aspiration is confirmed by lung re-expansion on repeat CXR. Occasionally intercostal chest drainage is required for a large PSP with respiratory failure or if aspiration is unsuccessful.

• In general, SP and traumatic pneumothoraces **always** require hospital admission and intercostal chest drain insertion (Fig. d). Multiple intercostal drains may be needed to ensure adequate lung re-expansion in some ICU patients with multiple loculated pneumothoraces. This strategy requires localization of airspaces on CT scan (Fig. c). High airways pressures and alveolar recruitment (e.g. CPAP or inverse ratio ventilation) encourage persistent leakage. 'Protective' ventilation and the lowest airway pressures compatible with adequate gas exchange should be used (Chapter 11). A persistent drain leak suggests development of a bronchopleural fistula (BPF). High flow, wall suction with pressures of 5–50 cmH_2O may oppose visceral and parietal pleura allowing spontaneous pleurodesis. Physiotherapy and bronchial toilette are required to maintain airway patency. Early advice on surgical BPF management is essential. Video-assisted thoracoscopy is as effective as thoracotomy at correcting BPF but causes less respiratory dysfunction.

• Chest drains are removed when CXR confirms lung expansion and there has been no air leakage through the drain for >24 h. Drains should not be clamped before removal. Following adequate analgesia, the drain is pulled out when the patient is in inspiration. Purse string sutures around the drainage site are then tightly secured.

Air leaks

Pneumomediastinum describes air in the mediastinal–pleural reflection, outlining the heart and great vessels on CXR. Air may also dissect along perivascular sheaths into the neck causing **subcutaneous emphysema (SE)** or around the heart with **pneumopericardium**, which may cause tamponade. Air leaks follow traumatic damage to the trachea (e.g. tracheostomy), bronchus and oesophagus (Chapter 46) or ventilator-induced barotrauma. SE may cause localized cervical or grotesque facial and body swelling. It has a characteristic crackling sensation on palpation. The voice may have a nasal quality and auscultation over the precordium may reveal a 'crunch' with each heart beat (Homan's sign). Management includes good drainage of pneumothorax and 'protective' ventilation strategies (Chapters 10, 11). Failure of spontaneous resolution should prompt investigation, including bronchoscopy, for problems that decrease chest drain efficiency or undetected air leaks.

(a) Patient positioning during massive haemoptysis

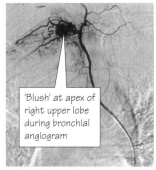

Promote drainage by:
• head down (Trendelenburg)
• lateral decubitus position

'Soiling' of 'good' uppermost lung is prevented by gravitational drainage. Thus, gas exchange is preserved

Presumed bleeding side of the chest is dependent to prevent soiling of unaffected lung

(b) The Heimlich manoeuvre for expulsion of an aspirated foreign body. Follow steps 1-3

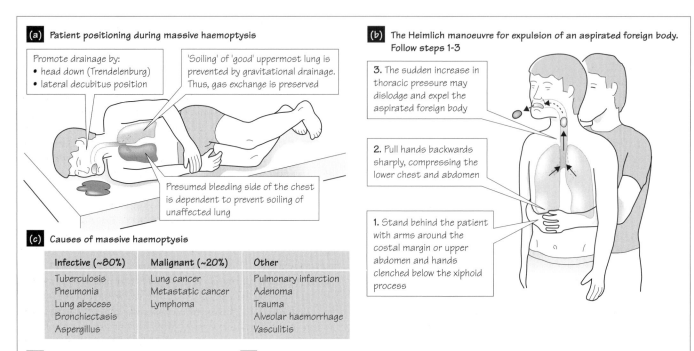

3. The sudden increase in thoracic pressure may dislodge and expel the aspirated foreign body

2. Pull hands backwards sharply, compressing the lower chest and abdomen

1. Stand behind the patient with arms around the costal margin or upper abdomen and hands clenched below the xiphoid process

(c) Causes of massive haemoptysis

Infective (~80%)	Malignant (~20%)	Other
Tuberculosis	Lung cancer	Pulmonary infarction
Pneumonia	Metastatic cancer	Adenoma
Lung abscess	Lymphoma	Trauma
Bronchiectasis		Alveolar haemorrhage
Aspergillus		Vasculitis

(d) Bronchial angiogram showing a localized area of bleeding

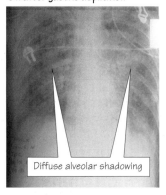

'Blush' at apex of right upper lobe during bronchial angiogram

(e) CXR of aspiration pneumonia occurring 6 h after gastric aspiration

Diffuse alveolar shadowing

(f) Diseases that may present as respiratory emergencies. Also see neuromuscular, endocrine and neurological chapters 23-28, 33, 37-40

Cause	Comments
CNS depression Coma (e.g. metabolic) CVA Sedation, self-poisoning	Perioperative sedation (e.g. benzodiazepines), self-poisoning (e.g. opiates) and strokes are associated with respiratory failure due to: • high risk of aspiration • loss of respiratory drive
Neurological diseases Myasthenia gravis Guillain-Barre syndrome* Restrictive wall defects (e.g. kyphoscoliosis) Myopathies Motor neurone disease	Require close monitoring as sudden respiratory failure may occur. Other problems include: • progressive respiratory muscle weakness • inadequate cough • atelectasis due to loss of mobility • laryngeal incompetence with aspiration
Infections Poliomyelitis Tetanus Diphtheria Botulism Tuberculosis (TB)	• Respiratory failure may develop within hours of polio infection. Bulbar lesions cause aspiration and pneumonia • A toxin-mediated disease due to *Clostridium tetani* causing muscle rigidity, spasms, respiratory failure, bulbar lesions + CVS instability • Respiratory failure is due to laryngeal obstruction by characteristic pharyngeal membrane or toxin-mediated polyneuritis • Potent neurotoxins produced by *Clostridium botulinum* inhibit presynaptic acetylcholine release causing respiratory failure • Acute respiratory failure occurs with massive haemoptysis or sudden rupture of pus into the bronchial tree with acute miliary TB
Endocrine disorders • Thyroid • Adrenal • Pituitary	Endocrine disorders can be complicated by respiratory failure due to CNS depression, muscle weakness or electrolyte imbalance

CNS=central nervous system, CVA=cerebrovascular accident, CVS=cardiovascular system

Massive haemoptysis
Definition. Expectoration of >600 mL of blood in 24 h.
Causes. Infection causes ~80% and malignancy <20% of cases (Fig. c).

Prognosis. Death is usually due to asphyxia, not blood loss, and is related to pathology, coexisting lung impairment and rate of bleeding (i.e. 600 mL haemoptysis over 4 h or 16 h causes 70% or 5% mortality, respectively).

Clinical evaluation. Haematemesis and nose bleeds are often confused with haemoptysis. Although food particles suggest haematemesis, expectorated blood is often swallowed. Purulent secretions suggest bronchiectasis or lung abscesses; apical cavities, tuberculosis or mycetoma; and haematuria, alveolar haemorrhage syndromes. Localization of the site of bleeding is difficult as aspiration results in diffuse clinical (e.g. crepitations) and radiological signs. **Investigations** include serology, blood gases, clotting profile, CXR and sputum microbiology (e.g. acid-fast bacilli).

Management involves:

1 *Protecting the airways.* Assess bleeding severity and institute measures to prevent asphyxia (e.g. oxygen therapy, secretion clearance). **Promote airways drainage** by placing the patient slightly head down in the lateral decubitus position (Fig. a). This prevents alveolar 'soiling' of the 'good' lung. Reduce bleeding by suppressing cough (e.g. codeine) and withholding physiotherapy. Indications for mechanical ventilation (MV) include overwhelming haemoptysis, respiratory distress and hypoxaemia. The unaffected lung can be independently ventilated by positioning the endotracheal tube in the corresponding main bronchus or by using a double-lumen tube until bleeding is controlled.

2 *Determine the site and cause of bleeding.* Early fibreoptic bronchoscopy allows examination of upper lobe and subsegmental bronchi, which account for ~80% of bleeding sites. Rigid bronchoscopy enhances suctioning in torrential haemorrhage but limits inspection. CT scans identify structural abnormalities (e.g. tumours) and bronchial arteriography, pulmonary angiography and nuclear scans may detect active bleeding (Fig. d).

3 *Control of bleeding.* Immediate measures include bronchoscopic iced saline (±adrenaline (epinephrine)) lavages, topical fibrin or tamponade of affected bronchi using balloon catheters.

• **Bronchial artery embolization** is initially successful in >70% of cases, especially those with dilated bronchial arteries (e.g. bronchiectasis). However, rebleeding is common (>50%) and serious complications occur including paraplegia following anterior spinal artery thrombosis (~5%).

• **Surgical therapy** has the best long-term outcomes but medical management is necessary in diffuse lesions or end-stage disease (e.g. cancer, $FEV_1 < 40\%$ of predicted).

4 *General measures,* including appropriate fluid replacement, antibiotics and bronchodilators.

Aspiration syndromes

High-risk groups for aspiration include those with depressed conscious level (e.g. drug overdose), laryngeal incompetence (e.g. bulbar syndromes) and critically ill patients. The clinical scenario depends on the type and volume of aspiration. Thus, perianaesthetic aspiration of large volumes of gastric contents rapidly progresses to ARDS, whereas repeated microaspiration (e.g. bulbar palsy) causes nosocomial pneumonia. A high index of suspicion is required as aspiration is not always witnessed.

• **Solid particulate matter** including peanuts, coins and teeth can be aspirated. Partially masticated food is most common, giving rise to the 'café coronary' syndrome. **Partial obstruction** causes stridor, cough, wheeze, atelectasis and recurrent pneumonia. **Complete obstruction** prevents breathing and speech with rapidly developing cyanosis, coma and death. If a sharp blow to the back of the chest fails to dislodge the particle, the Heimlich manoeuvre is attempted (Fig. b). If this fails, an emergency cricothyroidectomy is performed by inserting a large-bore needle or sharp implement through the cricothyroid membrane (Chapter 11). Urgent bronchoscopy follows to remove the obstruction.

• **Fluid aspiration.** Gastric contents (pH < 2) are most frequently aspirated. Significant volumes rapidly cause lung damage with respiratory failure, pulmonary oedema or ARDS. The right main bronchus is the most direct path and right lower lobe involvement is most common (~60%). Pulmonary infiltrates are seen on CXR in ~90% of cases (Fig. e). **Prevention is essential** (i.e. preoperative fasting, nasogastric tube drainage) as treatment is largely supportive including airways clearance, oxygen therapy, bronchodilators, antibiotics, CPAP or MV. Steroid therapy is not beneficial and bronchoscopy will not reduce damage. Nosocomial pneumonia due to microaspiration is prevented by semirecumbent nursing (i.e. >30° head-up) and early feeding which prevents gastric microbial overgrowth during stress ulcer prophylaxis.

• **Near-drowning** is a common cause of accidental death and is often associated with alcohol consumption or a primary medical event (e.g. MI). Although more frequent in river, sea or lakeside areas, deaths may occur at home in small volumes of water (e.g. bath). **Freshwater aspiration** affects pulmonary surfactant causing atelectasis, pulmonary shunt and hypoxaemia. Rapid absorption of hypotonic freshwater into the pulmonary circulation causes hypervolaemia, haemolysis and hyperkalaemia. Hypertonic **seawater aspiration** pulls fluid into alveoli causing hypovolaemia, shunting and hypoxaemia. Profound hypothermia (<30°C) is common in near-drowning and predisposes to resistant arrhythmias, particularly during rough handling (e.g. resuscitation). The Heimlich manoeuvre is not recommended as gravitational drainage of aspirated water is just as effective, without risking arrhythmias. Always rewarm hypothermic patients before terminating resuscitation (Chapter 21). Treatment is largely supportive and overnight observation is recommended as late pulmonary oedema can occur. The degree of hypoxic brain damage determines outcome (Chapter 45). Mortality is similar in fresh- or seawater.

Upper airways obstruction

Causes include aspirated particulate matter, inhaled toxic gases and burns (Chapter 49), trauma (Chapter 44, 46), anaphylaxis, laryngeal oedema, laryngospasm and large airway stenoses. Obstruction by the tongue should be excluded and prevented with a pharyngeal airway (Chapter 7). **Extubation** can be associated with laryngospasm due to upper airways stimulation during endotracheal tube removal or oedema. Severe respiratory distress requires immediate re-intubation. In less critical situations, nebulized adrenaline (epinephrine) and salbutamol with intravenous steroids may reduce oedema and spasm sufficiently to avoid re-intubation. **Helium and oxygen mixtures** may improve gas flow through upper airways obstruction.

Other respiratory emergencies

There is an extensive list of infective, neuromuscular and endocrine diseases (Chapters 23–28, 33, 37–40) that predispose to rapid respiratory impairment (Fig. f). Although rare in developed countries with advanced public health programmes, poliomyelitis, tetanus, diphtheria and tuberculosis remain relatively common causes of respiratory emergencies in the developing world.

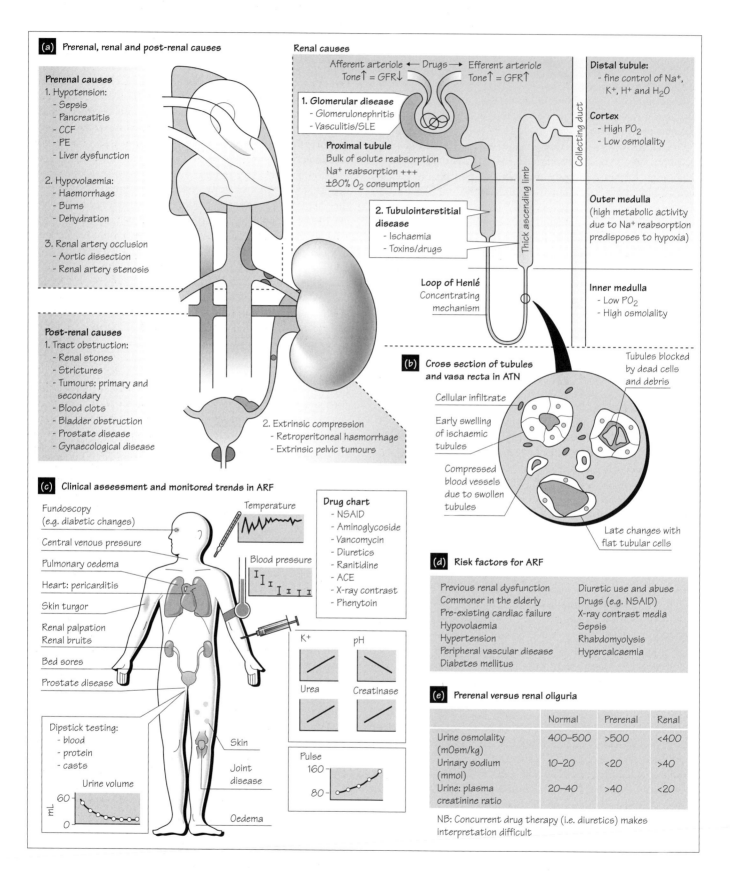

(a) Prerenal, renal and post-renal causes

Prerenal causes
1. Hypotension:
   - Sepsis
   - Pancreatitis
   - CCF
   - PE
   - Liver dysfunction

2. Hypovolaemia:
   - Haemorrhage
   - Burns
   - Dehydration

3. Renal artery occlusion
   - Aortic dissection
   - Renal artery stenosis

Post-renal causes
1. Tract obstruction:
   - Renal stones
   - Strictures
   - Tumours: primary and secondary
   - Blood clots
   - Bladder obstruction
   - Prostate disease
   - Gynaecological disease

2. Extrinsic compression
   - Retroperitoneal haemorrhage
   - Extrinsic pelvic tumours

Renal causes

Afferent arteriole ← Drugs → Efferent arteriole
Tone↑ = GFR↓   Tone↑ = GFR↑

1. Glomerular disease
   - Glomerulonephritis
   - Vasculitis/SLE

Proximal tubule
Bulk of solute reabsorption
Na$^+$ reabsorption +++
±80% O$_2$ consumption

2. Tubulointerstitial disease
   - Ischaemia
   - Toxins/drugs

Loop of Henlé
Concentrating mechanism

Thick ascending limb

Collecting duct

Distal tubule:
   - fine control of Na$^+$, K$^+$, H$^+$ and H$_2$O

Cortex
   - High PO$_2$
   - Low osmolality

Outer medulla
(high metabolic activity due to Na$^+$ reabsorption predisposes to hypoxia)

Inner medulla
   - Low PO$_2$
   - High osmolality

(b) Cross section of tubules and vasa recta in ATN

Cellular infiltrate

Early swelling of ischaemic tubules

Compressed blood vessels due to swollen tubules

Tubules blocked by dead cells and debris

Late changes with flat tubular cells

(c) Clinical assessment and monitored trends in ARF

Fundoscopy (e.g. diabetic changes)

Central venous pressure

Pulmonary oedema

Heart: pericarditis

Skin turgor

Renal palpation
Renal bruits

Bed sores

Prostate disease

Dipstick testing:
   - blood
   - protein
   - casts

Urine volume

Temperature

Blood pressure

Skin

Joint disease

Oedema

Drug chart
   - NSAID
   - Aminoglycoside
   - Vancomycin
   - Diuretics
   - Ranitidine
   - ACE
   - X-ray contrast
   - Phenytoin

K$^+$ pH

Urea   Creatinase

Pulse
160 –
80 –

(d) Risk factors for ARF

Previous renal dysfunction	Diuretic use and abuse
Commoner in the elderly	Drugs (e.g. NSAID)
Pre-existing cardiac failure	X-ray contrast media
Hypovolaemia	Sepsis
Hypertension	Rhabdomyolysis
Peripheral vascular disease	Hypercalcaemia
Diabetes mellitus	

(e) Prerenal versus renal oliguria

	Normal	Prerenal	Renal
Urine osmolality (mOsm/kg)	400–500	>500	<400
Urinary sodium (mmol)	10–20	<20	>40
Urine: plasma creatinine ratio	20–40	>40	<20

NB: Concurrent drug therapy (i.e. diuretics) makes interpretation difficult

Definition

Acute renal failure (ARF) is defined as sudden failure of the kidneys to excrete metabolic waste products, which subsequently accumulate in the blood (e.g. creatinine). It is often associated with a fall in glomerular filtration rate (GFR) and oliguria (reduced urine output; <400 mL daily) or anuria (no urine).

Classification of acute renal failure (Fig. a)

1 *Prerenal* (~55%) due to inadequate renal perfusion caused by hypotension (e.g. CCF, sepsis), circulatory volume depletion (e.g. haemorrhage) or renal blood supply obstruction. Resulting renal ischaemia may cause acute tubular necrosis (ATN).

2 *Renal* (~30%). Causes include:

- **Glomerular.** Glomerulonephritis, vasculitis, Goodpasture's syndrome.
- **Acute tubular necrosis and tubulointerstitial injury** caused by ischaemia, toxicity (e.g. drugs, heavy metals, contrast media) and free haemoglobin or myoglobin. Haemoglobin is released during haemolytic red cell destruction (e.g. haemolytic–uraemic syndrome) and myoglobin during rhabdomyolysis (e.g. trauma, muscle damage). ARF also follows tubular precipitation of myeloma light chains or calcium phosphate in acute hypercalcaemia.
- **Drugs and toxins.** NSAIDs cause renal arteriolar vasoconstriction by inhibiting normal prostaglandin-induced vasodilation. In hypovolaemic patients this seriously reduces renal blood flow and GFR. NSAIDs also contribute to ARF in patients with pre-existing renal impairment and those using diuretics (e.g. cirrhosis). Radiocontrasts, cyclosporin and amphotericin cause vasoconstriction, whereas aminoglycosides and cephalosporins are direct tubular toxins. ACE inhibitors block the angiotensin-mediated efferent arteriolar vasodilation that maintains GFR. Many drugs cause allergic tubulointerstitial nephritis (e.g. antibiotics, diuretics).

3 *Post-renal* (~15%) due to urinary tract obstruction (Fig. a). Resulting back-pressure inhibits GFR and causes ischaemia. ARF only occurs if both kidneys are obstructed.

Pathophysiology

Renal ischaemia contributes to most cases of ARF due to failure of the complex vascular control mechanisms. However, BP is a poor indicator of renal hypoperfusion as local arterial and tubuloglomerular autoregulatory feedback mechanisms act to maintain GFR and the renal renin–angiotensin mechanism raises BP despite hypovolaemia. The juxtamedullary region (i.e. proximal tubule and thick ascending limb of the loop of Henle) is particularly susceptible to ischaemia. This is because (i) active sodium absorption in this region accounts for 80% of renal oxygen consumption, and (ii) although the kidneys normally receive ~30% of cardiac output, the majority is directed to the cortex, whilst medullary blood flow is limited to maintain the concentration gradient of osmolality. Reduced renal blood flow (±sepsis, toxicity) causes ATN and tubular cell death in this region due to this combination of high oxygen demand and poor blood supply. Subsequent tubular blockage reduces GFR and swelling further compromises medullary perfusion (Fig. b).

Clinical features

There are two characteristic clinical presentations.

1 Most ARF occurs in critically ill patients (ICU incidence ~20–30%) and after surgery, trauma or burns as part of the multiple organ dysfunction syndrome ('**critical illness ARF**'). Although renal ischaemia (i.e. hypotension) is the main cause, aetiology is often multifactorial (i.e. sepsis, drugs). Presentation with oliguria and progressive increases in serum creatinine and urea (±metabolic acidosis, hyperkalaemia) is typical. Mortality is high (~40–60%) but renal function recovers (>85%) in most survivors. Long-term renal replacement therapy (RRT) is rarely required.

2 ARF occurring on the general ward due to specific renal diseases (e.g. glomerulonephritis) is less common ('**medical ARF**'). It usually presents as a failure to excrete nitrogenous waste rather than oliguria. Although mortality is low (~8%), it often progresses to chronic renal failure requiring RRT.

Clinical assessment (Fig. c)

The history identifies pre-existing factors which predispose to ARF (Table d). Haematuria or a recent throat or skin infection suggest glomerulonephritis. Haemoptysis is associated with Goodpasture's syndrome. Renal colic or male prostatism (e.g. frequency, poor stream) indicates post-renal obstruction. The past medical history may suggest possible associations (e.g. peripheral vascular disease (PVD) and renal artery stenosis; multisystem disease (e.g. SLE) and glomerulonephritis) and potential sites of chronic infection (e.g. endocarditis).

Examination

Examination must assess fluid status (i.e. is there hypovolaemia?), cardiovascular function (i.e. is there tissue hypoperfusion?) and PVD (i.e. is there a renal bruit?). Cardiac auscultation may reveal uraemic pericarditis or valve disease. The upper airways are examined for signs of Wegener's granulomatosis and the chest for pulmonary oedema. Abdominal examination may detect polycystic kidneys, bladder or prostatic enlargement and pelvic disease. Fundoscopy may identify diabetic or hypertensive changes. Sites of sepsis and features of multisystem disease (e.g. arthritis) must be sought.

- **Monitor** trends in: (i) **vital signs:** pulse, BP, CVP, urine output, fever and weight; (ii) **biochemical parameters:** potassium, urea, creatinine, calcium and pH. Creatine kinase indicates severity of rhabdomyolysis.
- **Investigations** include: **haematology** to assess anaemia and haemolysis; **urinalysis** to differentiate between hypovolaemia (prerenal) and renal failure (Table e); and **urine microscopy and culture:** Haematuria occurs in renal or post-renal disease. Haemoglobin indicates haemolysis. Proteinuria suggests glomerulonephritis or myeloma, and myoglobin rhabdomyolysis. Red cell casts are diagnostic of glomerulonephritis and granular casts occur in ATN. Urinary eosinophils suggest interstitial nephritis. **Microbiology** assesses urine, blood, chest and wound infections. **Immunology:** Antinuclear antibodies are high in SLE. Antiglomerular basement membrane antibody indicates Goodpasture's syndrome, and antineutrophil cytoplasmic antibodies (ANCA) suggest vasculitis (e.g. Wegener's). Low complement levels occur in SLE and postinfective glomerulonephritis. **Radiology:** Ultrasonography determines kidney size and excludes renal tract obstruction. Small kidneys indicate chronic renal disease. Radioisotope studies and angiography evaluate renal perfusion. **Histology:** Renal biopsy may be required to establish the cause of ARF.

Acute renal failure: pathophysiology and clinical aspects 69

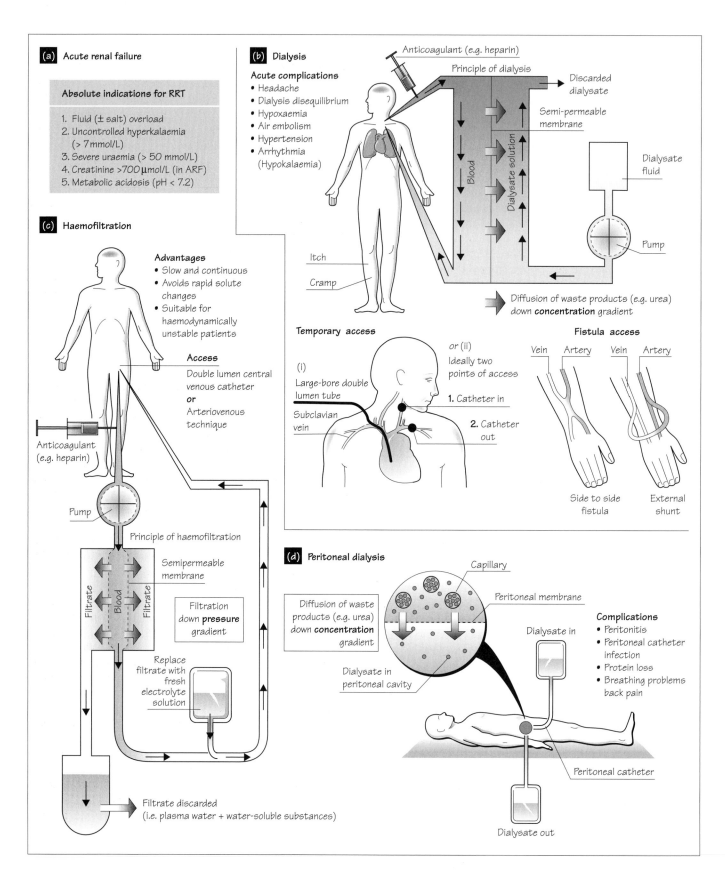

(a) Acute renal failure

Absolute indications for RRT

1. Fluid (± salt) overload
2. Uncontrolled hyperkalaemia (> 7 mmol/L)
3. Severe uraemia (> 50 mmol/L)
4. Creatinine >700 μmol/L (in ARF)
5. Metabolic acidosis (pH < 7.2)

(b) Dialysis

Acute complications
• Headache
• Dialysis disequilibrium
• Hypoxaemia
• Air embolism
• Hypertension
• Arrhythmia (Hypokalaemia)

Anticoagulant (e.g. heparin)

Principle of dialysis

Discarded dialysate

Semi-permeable membrane

Dialysate fluid

Blood

Dialysate solution

Pump

Itch

Cramp

Diffusion of waste products (e.g. urea) down **concentration** gradient

Temporary access

(i)
Large-bore double lumen tube

Subclavian vein

or (ii)
Ideally two points of access

1. Catheter in
2. Catheter out

Fistula access

Vein   Artery   Vein   Artery

Side to side fistula

External shunt

(c) Haemofiltration

Advantages
• Slow and continuous
• Avoids rapid solute changes
• Suitable for haemodynamically unstable patients

Access
Double lumen central venous catheter
or
Arteriovenous technique

Anticoagulant (e.g. heparin)

Pump

Principle of haemofiltration

Semipermeable membrane

Filtrate   Blood   Filtrate

Filtration down **pressure** gradient

Replace filtrate with fresh electrolyte solution

Filtrate discarded
(i.e. plasma water + water-soluble substances)

(d) Peritoneal dialysis

Diffusion of waste products (e.g. urea) down **concentration** gradient

Capillary

Peritoneal membrane

Dialysate in peritoneal cavity

Dialysate in

Complications
• Peritonitis
• Peritoneal catheter infection
• Protein loss
• Breathing problems back pain

Peritoneal catheter

Dialysate out

Prevention of acute renal failure (ARF)

A primary objective in the critically ill patient is to prevent ARF. Early recognition of oliguria and renal dysfunction allows institution of measures to reverse ischaemia/toxicity and re-establish urine output and renal function.

1 *Identify and treat the cause* including prerenal, renal and postrenal pathology (e.g. steroids for vasculitis).

2 *Fluid management.* Regular assessment of fluid and electrolyte balance is essential (Chapters 4, 5). Fluid intake, urine output and daily weight are monitored. A central venous catheter may be required to measure CVP. Volume replacement should match daily and insensible losses with an additional 0.5 L/°C of fever. Inadequate perfusion and renal ischaemia (e.g. hypovolaemia, hypotension) are the commonest causes of ARF and *must be corrected immediately.* If oliguria or renal dysfunction (i.e. rising urea or creatinine concentrations) develops, consider the following.

- **Fluid challenge** (~0.5–1 L NS over 30–60 min) particularly if clinical examination (±urinalysis) indicates a prerenal cause. The aim is to raise CVP, BP and GFR. Increased urine output supports the diagnosis. Further fluid challenges are guided by CVP assessment. In established ATN or intrinsic renal disease, oliguria will persist and continued fluid administration risks pulmonary oedema.
- **Diuretics.** Frusemide inhibits sodium absorption in the loop of Henle and the associated reduction in oxygen consumption has potential tubuloprotective effects. Continuous frusemide infusions (2–10 mg/h) or intermittent doses (80–250 mg over 1–4 h) are often recommended but despite increased urine production there is little evidence that ARF is prevented. In hypovolaemic patients, frusemide causes nephro-/ototoxicity and potentiates drug toxicity (e.g. aminoglycosides). It should be discontinued if urine output does not increase within 8 h. The osmotic diuretic mannitol has no additional benefit except with urine alkalinization in rhabdomyolysis.
- **Inotropes** (e.g. adrenaline) maintain GFR by increasing cardiac output and MAP (i.e. >70 mmHg) if fluid resuscitation is unsuccessful.
- **Low-dose 'renal' dopamine** has diuretic effects but its use in ARF is controversial due to potential adverse effects (e.g. arrhythmias). Prophylactic benefit is unproven.

3 *Oxygenation.* Optimize gas exchange (Chapter 6).

4 *Sepsis* must be identified and treated (e.g. antibiotics, surgery).

5 *Monitor biochemistry and drug levels.* Correct electrolyte imbalance/acidosis and adjust prescriptions.

6 *Renal protection* (e.g. N-acetylcysteine for radioisotopes).

Established acute renal failure (ERF)

Once ARF is established, treatment is supportive. Management aims to (i) prevent fluid overload, (ii) maintain electrolyte and acid–base balance, and (iii) limit accumulation of toxic metabolic waste by nutritional control and RRT. In patients with ATN, spontaneous recovery of renal function occurs after ~5–20 days (range 2–60 days) and is heralded by a diuretic phase. ERF due to other causes may be associated with persisting renal dysfunction and the need for ongoing renal support.

General management

- **Fluid balance.** During anuric or oliguric periods, fluid replacement is restricted to insensible loss (~1 L/day). If pulmonary oedema occurs due to fluid overload (Chapter 20), it is treated with oxygen and pulmonary vasodilators (e.g. nitrates, opiates) whilst RRT is arranged to remove fluid. CPAP and venesection may help. During the diuretic phase of ATN recovery, fluid losses and electrolyte imbalance must be corrected.
- **Electrolytes** are monitored daily and sodium and potassium intake restricted. Calcium exchange resins, insulin with dextrose or RRT may be required to prevent hyperkalaemia. During ERF serum creatinine rises by ~80–100 μmol/L/day but this depends on muscle mass, metabolic rate and tissue damage. The rate of rise of urea is more variable. Serious uraemic complications (e.g. pericarditis, seizures, vomiting) develop above 50 mmol/L.
- **Diet.** A high-carbohydrate diet (2000–3000 calories) minimizes body protein catabolism. Protein intake <40–50 g/day reduces nitrogenous waste production.
- **Metabolic acidosis** is initially corrected by hyperventilation and compensatory hypocapnia. Respiratory distress and myocardial instability are indications for RRT.
- **Anaemia and bleeding** due to uraemia are corrected with blood and clotting factors.
- **General factors.** Modify drug doses, control hypertension and prevent infection (e.g. line sepsis). Remove urinary catheters in anuric patients.

Renal replacement therapy

Absolute indications for RRT are listed in Fig. (a). Three main methods of fluid and solute removal are used in ERF.

- **Dialysis** (Fig. b). Blood flows on one side and a solution of crystalloids (dialysis fluid) is pumped in the opposite direction along the other side of a semipermeable membrane. Small molecules and toxic waste diffuse across the membrane according to imposed concentration gradients. Dialysis fluid composition is designed to normalize plasma. Small molecules such as urea (60 Da) are efficiently removed, larger molecules like creatinine (113 Da) less so. Hyperphosphataemia due to poor clearance of phosphate ions occurs during intermittent dialysis. Dialysis corrects biochemical abnormalities and removes accumulated extracellular fluid rapidly (~2–4 h) but may cause hypovolaemia or hypokalaemia. In haemodynamically unstable patients, life-threatening hypotension or cardiac arrhythmias may occur.
- **Haemofiltration** (Fig. c). Plasma water and water-soluble substances (molecular weight <20 kDa) pass across a highly permeable membrane by convective flow (e.g. glomerular filtration). Unlike dialysis, urea, creatinine and phosphate are cleared at similar rates. Hypophosphataemia may occur if phosphate is not supplemented. Molecules like heparin are also efficiently cleared. The filtrate is discarded and replaced by a physiological solution. Low flow rates make haemofiltration less efficient at removing uraemic toxins but continuous use allows clearance of any amount of fluid and nitrogenous waste. Haemofiltration's advantage is relative ease of use in haemodynamically unstable patients.
- **Peritoneal dialysis** (Fig. d) uses hypertonic dialysate to draw fluid and solutes across the peritoneum following insertion of a peritoneal catheter. The dialysate (1–3 L) dwells in the abdominal cavity for ~30–40 min before drainage. In critically ill patients, infection risks and interference with ventilation limit use. It cannot be used in patients with abdominal pathology.

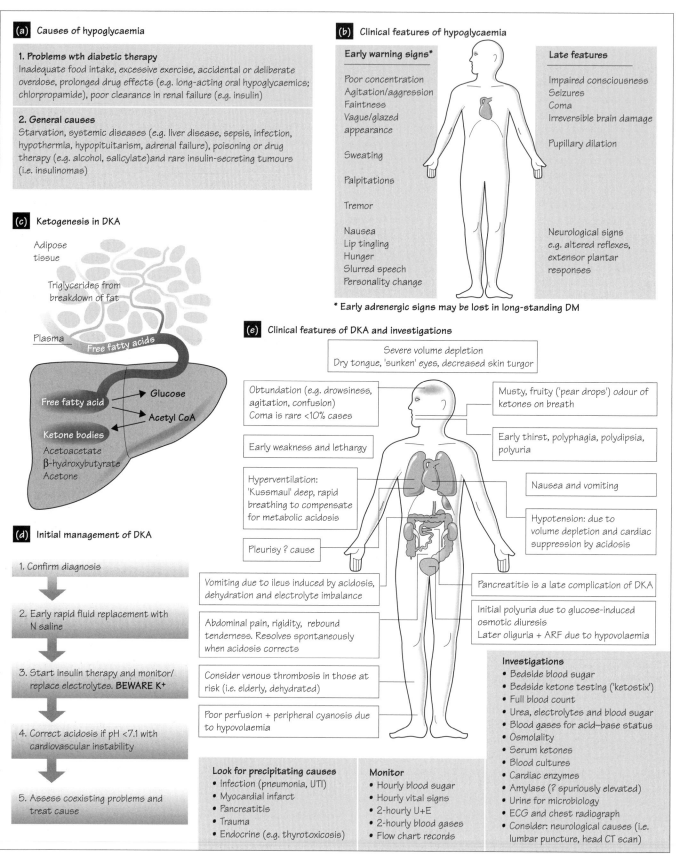

(a) Causes of hypoglycaemia

1. Problems wth diabetic therapy
Inadequate food intake, excessive exercise, accidental or deliberate overdose, prolonged drug effects (e.g. long-acting oral hypoglycaemics; chlorpropamide), poor clearance in renal failure (e.g. insulin)

2. General causes
Starvation, systemic diseases (e.g. liver disease, sepsis, infection, hypothermia, hypopituitarism, adrenal failure), poisoning or drug therapy (e.g. alcohol, salicylate) and rare insulin-secreting tumours (i.e. insulinomas)

(b) Clinical features of hypoglycaemia

Early warning signs*

Poor concentration
Agitation/aggression
Faintness
Vague/glazed appearance

Sweating

Palpitations

Tremor

Nausea
Lip tingling
Hunger
Slurred speech
Personality change

Late features

Impaired consciousness
Seizures
Coma
Irreversible brain damage

Pupillary dilation

Neurological signs e.g. altered reflexes, extensor plantar responses

* Early adrenergic signs may be lost in long-standing DM

(c) Ketogenesis in DKA

Adipose tissue

Triglycerides from breakdown of fat

Plasma
Free fatty acids

Free fatty acid → Glucose
→ Acetyl CoA
Ketone bodies
Acetoacetate
β-hydroxybutyrate
Acetone

(d) Initial management of DKA

1. Confirm diagnosis

2. Early rapid fluid replacement with N saline

3. Start insulin therapy and monitor/ replace electrolytes. BEWARE K+

4. Correct acidosis if pH <7.1 with cardiovascular instability

5. Assess coexisting problems and treat cause

(e) Clinical features of DKA and investigations

Severe volume depletion
Dry tongue, 'sunken' eyes, decreased skin turgor

Obtundation (e.g. drowsiness, agitation, confusion) Coma is rare <10% cases

Musty, fruity ('pear drops') odour of ketones on breath

Early weakness and lethargy

Early thirst, polyphagia, polydipsia, polyuria

Hyperventilation: 'Kussmaul' deep, rapid breathing to compensate for metabolic acidosis

Nausea and vomiting

Pleurisy ? cause

Hypotension: due to volume depletion and cardiac suppression by acidosis

Vomiting due to ileus induced by acidosis, dehydration and electrolyte imbalance

Pancreatitis is a late complication of DKA

Abdominal pain, rigidity, rebound tenderness. Resolves spontaneously when acidosis corrects

Initial polyuria due to glucose-induced osmotic diuresis
Later oliguria + ARF due to hypovolaemia

Consider venous thrombosis in those at risk (i.e. elderly, dehydrated)

Poor perfusion + peripheral cyanosis due to hypovolaemia

Investigations
• Bedside blood sugar
• Bedside ketone testing ('ketostix')
• Full blood count
• Urea, electrolytes and blood sugar
• Blood gases for acid–base status
• Osmolality
• Serum ketones
• Blood cultures
• Cardiac enzymes
• Amylase (? spuriously elevated)
• Urine for microbiology
• ECG and chest radiograph
• Consider: neurological causes (i.e. lumbar puncture, head CT scan)

Look for precipitating causes
• Infection (pneumonia, UTI)
• Myocardial infarct
• Pancreatitis
• Trauma
• Endocrine (e.g. thyrotoxicosis)

Monitor
• Hourly blood sugar
• Hourly vital signs
• 2-hourly U+E
• 2-hourly blood gases
• Flow chart records

Diabetes mellitus (DM) is a metabolic disorder characterized by hyperglycaemia (blood sugar (BS) > 11.1 mmol/L) due to a deficiency of, or resistance to, insulin.

- **Type I DM** usually presents in young people (<30 years). Genetic (HLA-linked), autoimmune and viral factors contribute to pancreatic β-islet cell destruction and insulin deficiency. Hyperglycaemic symptoms (e.g. polyuria, weight loss, fatigue) progress to ketoacidosis if insulin therapy is not commenced.
- **Type II DM** occurs in older adults (>40 years) with insulin resistance (± impaired production). There is a strong genetic association but diet and obesity determine age of onset. Treatment is with diet ± oral hypoglycaemic agents including biguanides (e.g. metformin) and/or sulphonylureas (e.g. gliclazide). Insulin therapy is required if BS control is poor and during intercurrent illness.
- **Other causes of DM** include malnutrition and secondary DM (e.g. pancreatitis, endocrine disease, steroids).
- **Stress-induced hyperglycaemia** may occur in any critically ill patient. Tight glycaemic control with insulin infusions improves outcome.

In critical care units DM presents as end-organ damage (e.g. nephropathy) or life-threatening diabetic emergencies (see below).

Hypoglycaemia

Hypoglycaemia occurs when BS is <4 mmol/L, but the symptom threshold varies. It must be suspected in every patient with sudden changes in mental state or neurological function. **Causes** are listed in Fig. (a). Problems with diabetic therapy are most common.

Clinical features (Fig. b) include early 'adrenergic' symptoms (e.g. tremor, sweating), followed by progressive confusion and seizures. Coma and irreversible neurological damage rapidly follow due to the brain's dependence on glucose metabolism.

Management. Bedside BS measurement confirms hypoglycaemia. A glucose drink or 'carbohydrate snack' is given to conscious patients and intravenous glucose (e.g. 50–100 mL 20% dextrose) when the conscious level is depressed. Severe or refractory hypoglycaemia (e.g. sulphonylurea overdose) may require glucagon or hydrocortisone therapy and these patients must be admitted for BS monitoring (± glucose infusions). When BS measurement is unavailable, glucose may have to be given empirically. Supplemental thiamine prevents Wernicke's encephalopathy (i.e. eye movement paralysis, ataxia, confusion) in malnourished patients (e.g. alcoholics).

Diabetic ketoacidosis (DKA)

DKA occurs in type I DM. Despite aggressive therapy mortality is ~5%. Precipitating factors include infection (~30%), MI and pancreatitis. No cause is found in ~25%. **Pathogenesis:** Insulin deficiency and stress hormones accelerate hepatic glucose production and prevent cellular glucose uptake. Resulting hyperglycaemia (BS ~20–40 mmol/L) exceeds the renal glucose threshold and glycosuria causes an osmotic diuresis with water and electrolyte loss. Dehydration occurs when nausea and vomiting prevent adequate fluid intake. Similar hormonal changes cause intracellular lipolysis. Hepatic metabolism of released fatty acids results in ketone production (e.g. α-hydroxybutyrate) and metabolic acidosis (Fig. c).

Clinical presentation (Fig. e). ~10% of type I DM presents as DKA. Nausea, lethargy, thirst and polyuria often precede DKA, which may develop within hours. Presenting features are due to **severe volume depletion** (e.g. hypotension, hypoperfusion) and **metabolic acidosis** (e.g. hyperventilation).

Investigation (Fig. e). Bedside BS testing and urinary ketones confirm the diagnosis. Laboratory tests assess dehydration, electrolyte imbalance and acidosis. The precipitating cause and coexisting problems (e.g. renal failure) must be established.

Management (Fig. d). Haemodynamic instability due to severe volume depletion (±acidosis) and rapid ion fluxes during initial therapy (particularly K^+) are potentially lethal.

- **Resuscitation.** Immediate fluid therapy with normal saline rapidly corrects hypovolaemia and restores cardiovascular stability (i.e. 1 L in 30 min, then 1 L over 1 h, etc.). Total fluid deficits of ~5–10 L and sodium losses of ~400 mmol are replaced over 24–48 h. Monitor CVP if pulmonary oedema is a risk.
- **Insulin infusion,** initially at 6 U/h (with hourly BS monitoring) aims to reduce BS by 3–5 mmol/h. Osmotic shifts during rapid BS correction can cause cerebral oedema.
- **Electrolyte replacement.** Diuresis (±vomiting) cause severe potassium (K^+) depletion. However, initial serum K^+ levels are high due to acidosis-induced K^+ shift from the intracellular to extracellular space. Insulin therapy and correction of acidosis stimulate cellular K^+ uptake and serum K^+ levels rapidly fall. Hourly monitoring and K^+ supplements (20–80 mmol/h) prevent severe hypokalaemia and cardiac arrest. Hypomagnesaemia is corrected to prevent insulin resistance and arrhythmias. Phosphate supplements maintain tissue oxygenation.
- **Correct acidosis.** Fluid and insulin therapy reverse acidosis within hours. Sodium bicarbonate therapy is controversial. It may reduce oxygen delivery and cause hypokalaemia. However, in severe acidosis (pH < 7.1) with myocardial depression treatment may be unavoidable.
- **General measures** include supplemental oxygen, antibiotics and nasogastric tube drainage to prevent aspiration (e.g. coma).
- **The postresuscitation phase** is often poorly managed and a diabetic specialist should be involved. When BS is <10 mmol/L, a 5% dextrose infusion is commenced. Regular insulin regimes restart when ketoacidosis resolves and nutrition is normal.

Hyperosmolar non-ketotic coma (HONK)

HONK is less common than DKA but mortality is ~50%. It occurs in elderly type II DM with sufficient insulin production to prevent ketogenesis but not hyperglycaemia. Osmotic diuresis leads to severe dehydration and hyperosmolality. Metabolic acidosis does not occur.

Clinical features. Anorexia, malaise, polyuria and weakness progress slowly to confusion, seizures and coma. Diagnosis is based on BS (>40 mmol/L) and hyperosmolality (>330 mOsm/L). Serum sodium is often >160 mmol/L.

Management. Rehydration with normal saline should be slower than in DKA despite greater fluid deficits. Gradual sodium and BS reductions (e.g. low-dose insulin) avoid sudden osmotic and electrolyte shifts, which may precipitate cerebral oedema and central pontine demyelinolysis. Anticoagulation is essential to prevent dehydration-induced thromboembolic events.

Lactic acidosis

Lactic acidosis occurs in type II DM treated with metformin. Despite bicarbonate therapy, prognosis is poor.

33 Endocrine emergencies

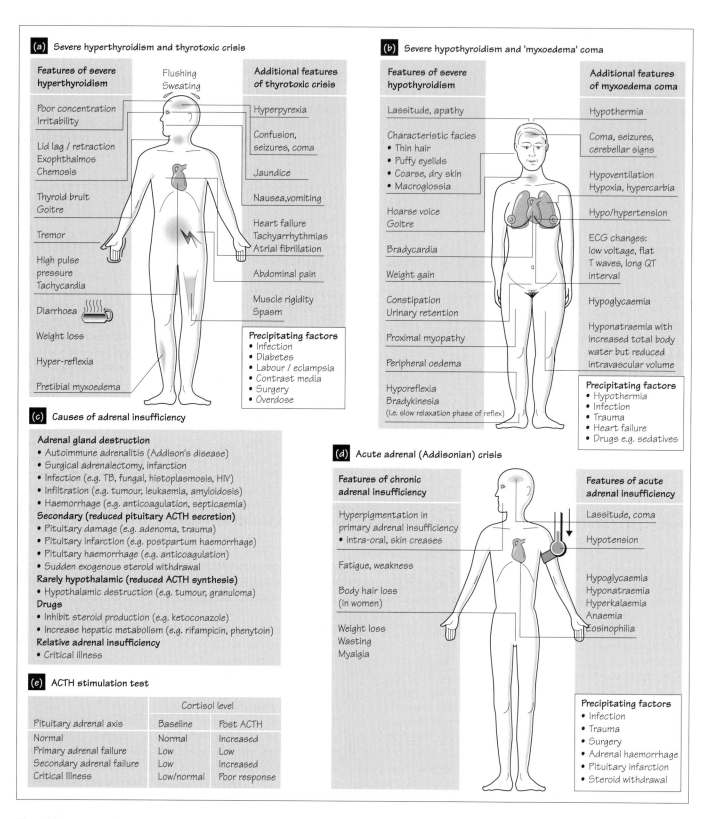

(a) Severe hyperthyroidism and thyrotoxic crisis

Features of severe hyperthyroidism

Poor concentration
Irritability

Lid lag / retraction
Exophthalmos
Chemosis

Thyroid bruit
Goitre

Tremor

High pulse pressure
Tachycardia

Diarrhoea

Weight loss

Hyper-reflexia

Pretibial myxoedema

Flushing
Sweating

Additional features of thyrotoxic crisis

Hyperpyrexia

Confusion, seizures, coma

Jaundice

Nausea, vomiting

Heart failure
Tachyarrhythmias
Atrial fibrillation

Abdominal pain

Muscle rigidity
Spasm

Precipitating factors
• Infection
• Diabetes
• Labour / eclampsia
• Contrast media
• Surgery
• Overdose

(b) Severe hypothyroidism and 'myxoedema' coma

Features of severe hypothyroidism

Lassitude, apathy

Characteristic facies
• Thin hair
• Puffy eyelids
• Coarse, dry skin
• Macroglossia

Hoarse voice
Goitre

Bradycardia

Weight gain

Constipation
Urinary retention

Proximal myopathy

Peripheral oedema

Hyporeflexia
Bradykinesia
(i.e. slow relaxation phase of reflex)

Additional features of myxoedema coma

Hypothermia

Coma, seizures, cerebellar signs

Hypoventilation
Hypoxia, hypercarbia

Hypo/hypertension

ECG changes: low voltage, flat T waves, long QT interval

Hypoglycaemia

Hyponatraemia with increased total body water but reduced intravascular volume

Precipitating factors
• Hypothermia
• Infection
• Trauma
• Heart failure
• Drugs e.g. sedatives

(c) Causes of adrenal insufficiency

Adrenal gland destruction
• Autoimmune adrenalitis (Addison's disease)
• Surgical adrenalectomy, infarction
• Infection (e.g. TB, fungal, histoplasmosis, HIV)
• Infiltration (e.g. tumour, leukaemia, amyloidosis)
• Haemorrhage (e.g. anticoagulation, septicaemia)
Secondary (reduced pituitary ACTH secretion)
• Pituitary damage (e.g. adenoma, trauma)
• Pituitary infarction (e.g. postpartum haemorrhage)
• Pituitary haemorrhage (e.g. anticoagulation)
• Sudden exogenous steroid withdrawal
Rarely hypothalamic (reduced ACTH synthesis)
• Hypothalamic destruction (e.g. tumour, granuloma)
Drugs
• Inhibit steroid production (e.g. ketoconazole)
• Increase hepatic metabolism (e.g. rifampicin, phenytoin)
Relative adrenal insufficiency
• Critical illness

(d) Acute adrenal (Addisonian) crisis

Features of chronic adrenal insufficiency

Hyperpigmentation in primary adrenal insufficiency
• intra-oral, skin creases

Fatigue, weakness

Body hair loss (in women)

Weight loss
Wasting
Myalgia

Features of acute adrenal insufficiency

Lassitude, coma

Hypotension

Hypoglycaemia
Hyponatraemia
Hyperkalaemia
Anaemia
Eosinophilia

Precipitating factors
• Infection
• Trauma
• Surgery
• Adrenal haemorrhage
• Pituitary infarction
• Steroid withdrawal

(e) ACTH stimulation test

Pituitary adrenal axis	Cortisol level	
	Baseline	Post ACTH
Normal	Normal	Increased
Primary adrenal failure	Low	Low
Secondary adrenal failure	Low	Increased
Critical Illness	Low/normal	Poor response

Thyroid emergencies
• Thyrotoxic crisis is a life-threatening hypermetabolic emergency in which the characteristics of hyperthyroidism are accentuated. It is precipitated by infection, surgery, diabetes, labour, radioiodine therapy and iodinated contrast media. Thyroxine overdose and eclampsia are occasional causes. Mortality is ~25%.

Clinical features (Fig. a). No absolute signs differentiate thyrotoxic crisis from severe hyperthyroidism. High-output cardiac failure complicates ~50% of cases. Differential diagnosis includes sepsis, phaeochromocytoma, drug abuse and malignant hyperthermia.

General management. Identify and treat the precipitating cause. Correct dehydration and electrolyte disturbances. Institute cooling but avoid aspirin, which displaces thyroid hormone from binding protein. Sedation reduces agitation and dantrolene relieves the effects of extreme muscle activity.

Specific therapy includes:

Beta-blockade which inhibits the peripheral effects of thyroid hormone, reducing heart rate, hypertension, fever and tremor.

Thiourea derivatives which block T4 synthesis. Propylthiouracil is preferred because it blocks T4 to T3 conversion but it must be given enterally. Carbimazole is metabolized to methimazole and, although onset is slower, its action is longer and it can be given by rectal suppository. White cell suppression occurs with both drugs and therapy is stopped if a sore throat develops.

Prevention of T4 release which is achieved with iodine solutions, lithium or dexamethasone. Iodine inhibits thyroid uptake of thiourea. Consequently, thioureas **must** be administered 2 h before iodine to prevent thyrotoxic crisis.

• **Severe hypothyroidism (myxoedema coma)** is manifest when intercurrent illness (e.g. infection) or drugs (e.g. sedatives) complicate pre-existing hypothyroidism causing hypothermia, coma and hypotension. It usually affects elderly females with unrecognized hypothyroidism due to auto-immune thyroiditis, thyroidectomy, radioiodine or drug therapy (e.g. amiodarone) or patients who fail to take replacement thyroxine. Mortality is high.

Clinical features (Fig. b) are those of severe hypothyroidism.

Investigation may reveal anaemia, hypoglycaemia, hyponatraemia, hypophosphataemia and ECG changes (Fig. b). In primary hypothyroidism, thyroid-stimulating hormone (TSH) is raised and T3/T4 low. In pituitary failure both TSH and T3/T4 are low.

Management includes rewarming, respiratory support and correction of hypoglycaemia. Intravenous thyroxine (T4) is given in slowly increasing doses. Concurrent adrenal insufficiency may occur and until excluded corticosteroid therapy is required.

• **Sick euthyroid syndrome** is often detected in critical illness. It is not due to a thyroid disorder and should not be treated. Low T4 binding protein and altered T4 metabolism result in abnormal thyroid function tests (e.g. low total T4, normal free T4, low T3 and normal TSH levels).

Adrenal emergencies

• **Adrenocortical insufficiency (AI)** describes reduced cortisol (±aldosterone) production by the adrenal cortex.

Causes are listed in Fig. (c). Primary adrenal insufficiency (PAI) follows adrenal damage (e.g. autoimmune adrenalitis; 'Addison's disease'). Secondary adrenal insufficiency (SAI) due to adrenocorticotrophic hormone (ACTH) deficiency follows pituitary or hypothalamic damage. Abrupt withdrawal of therapeutic steroids may also present as AI because ACTH secretion remains depressed after clearance of exogenous steroid.

Clinical presentation (Fig. d) is either acute or chronic.

Acute (Addisonian) crises are precipitated by stress (e.g. surgery) in patients with unrecognized chronic AI or following sepsis or adrenal haemorrhage during critical illness. Pituitary infarction after postpartum haemorrhage (Sheehan's syndrome) also presents as acute AI. Characteristic features are apathy, hypoglycaemia, hypotension (±shock) and coma. The diagnosis should be suspected in all patients with shock if the cause is not apparent. In critical illness, relative AI is common (i.e. ACTH stimulation produces only small increases in high baseline cortisol levels). These patients may benefit from steroid supplementation.

Chronic deficiency (e.g. autoimmune adrenalitis) presents with fatigue, weakness, weight loss, fever and nausea. In PAI, hyperpigmentation is caused by excess pituitary melanocyte-stimulating hormone. Body hair loss in females is due to reduced adrenal androgen production.

Investigation. Hyponatraemia and hyperkalaemia are features of aldosterone reduction in PAI. Hypoglycaemia, hypercalcaemia, eosinophilia and volume depletion with raised blood urea occur in all forms of AI. Immunology may reveal auto-antibodies. **Adrenal function tests** must not delay cortisol replacement. A low baseline cortisol confirms AI. Cortisol levels taken 30 and 60 min after intravenous ACTH injection often indicate the cause (Fig. e). ACTH is high in PAI and low in SAI.

Treatment of shock (Chapters 4, 5) may require aggressive fluid therapy (e.g. 6 L NS over 24 h) and inotropic support. High-dose corticosteroids are needed because stress increases baseline cortisol levels by ~10-fold. Dexamethasone does not interfere with serum cortisol assays. Hyperkalaemia corrects rapidly with fluid and steroids. Treat infection with antibiotics and hypoglycaemia with glucose supplements.

• **Adrenocortical excess.** Cortisol is increased in Cushing's syndrome (e.g. steroid therapy, adrenal tumours) and Cushing's disease (e.g. ACTH-secreting pituitary tumour). Characteristic features include a moon face, thin easily bruised skin, hypertension (~50%), diabetes (~10%), osteoporosis (~50%), central obesity and hypokalaemia (e.g. arrhythmias, muscle weakness). Excess aldosterone secretion from an adrenal adenoma (Conn's syndrome) causes hypokalaemia, muscle weakness (e.g. postoperative ventilatory impairment) and hypertension.

Other endocrine emergencies

• **Hypopituitary crisis** follows pituitary trauma, infiltration (e.g. tumour), haemorrhage or infarction. Reduced anterior pituitary hormone secretion causes adrenal and thyroid insufficiency (see above) and hypogonadism. Failure of posterior pituitary antidiuretic hormone release causes diabetes insipidus with thirst, dehydration and severe polyuria. Detailed assessment of the pituitary–adrenal axis and hormone replacement therapy are required.

• **Phaeochromocytomas** are rare, benign (~90%), adrenal (~90%) tumours that release catecholamines. They are often familial and associated with other tumours (e.g. multiple endocrine neoplasia). Crises can be precipitated by drugs, surgery and foods (e.g. cheese). Features include headaches, sweating, flushing and arrhythmias. Hypertension may be sustained or labile. Raised plasma catecholamines or 24-h urinary vanillyl mandelic acid (VMA) confirm the diagnosis. Treatment is with α-blockers (e.g. phenoxybenzamine), β-blockers and surgery.

34 Gastrointestinal haemorrhage

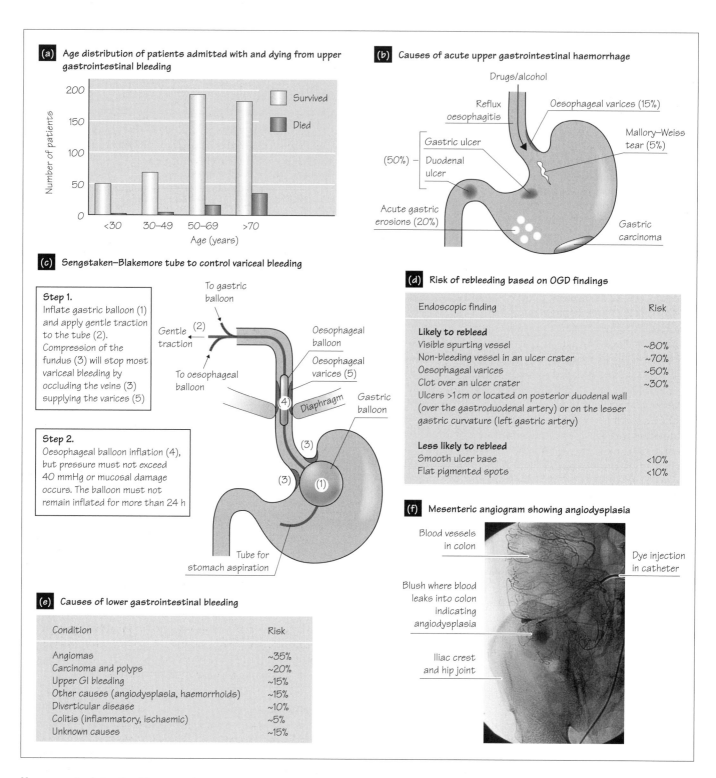

(a) Age distribution of patients admitted with and dying from upper gastrointestinal bleeding

(b) Causes of acute upper gastrointestinal haemorrhage

Drugs/alcohol
Reflux oesophagitis
Oesophageal varices (15%)
Mallory–Weiss tear (5%)
Gastric ulcer
Duodenal ulcer
(50%)
Acute gastric erosions (20%)
Gastric carcinoma

(c) Sengstaken–Blakemore tube to control variceal bleeding

Step 1.
Inflate gastric balloon (1) and apply gentle traction to the tube (2). Compression of the fundus (3) will stop most variceal bleeding by occluding the veins (3) supplying the varices (5)

Step 2.
Oesophageal balloon inflation (4), but pressure must not exceed 40 mmHg or mucosal damage occurs. The balloon must not remain inflated for more than 24 h

To gastric balloon
Gentle traction (2)
To oesophageal balloon
Oesophageal balloon
Oesophageal varices (5)
(4)
Diaphragm
Gastric balloon
(3)
(3)
(1)
Tube for stomach aspiration

(d) Risk of rebleeding based on OGD findings

Endoscopic finding	Risk
Likely to rebleed	
Visible spurting vessel	~80%
Non-bleeding vessel in an ulcer crater	~70%
Oesophageal varices	~50%
Clot over an ulcer crater	~30%
Ulcers >1cm or located on posterior duodenal wall (over the gastroduodenal artery) or on the lesser gastric curvature (left gastric artery)	
Less likely to rebleed	
Smooth ulcer base	<10%
Flat pigmented spots	<10%

(f) Mesenteric angiogram showing angiodysplasia

Blood vessels in colon
Dye injection in catheter
Blush where blood leaks into colon indicating angiodysplasia
Iliac crest and hip joint

(e) Causes of lower gastrointestinal bleeding

Condition	Risk
Angiomas	~35%
Carcinoma and polyps	~20%
Upper GI bleeding	~15%
Other causes (angiodysplasia, haemorrhoids)	~15%
Diverticular disease	~10%
Colitis (inflammatory, ischaemic)	~5%
Unknown causes	~15%

Upper gastrointestinal haemorrhage

Incidence. Acute upper GI bleeding affects ~1/1000 population and is most common in patients >50 years old (Fig. a). Significant bleeding due to stress ulceration occurs in <10% of critically ill patients. **Causes** (Fig. b) include peptic ulceration (~50%), gastritis/oesophagitis (20%) and oesophageal varices (15%). No cause is found in ~20%. Aspirin and NSAIDs cause gastritis and ulceration. Cirrhosis is the commonest cause of portal hypertension (PrHT) and oesophageal varices develop when portal pressure is >12mmHg. Acute variceal bleeding occurs in ~30% and accounts for >70% of upper GI bleeds in cirrhotics.

Clinical features

Most patients present with haematemesis (i.e. vomited fresh or altered blood; ~50–65%), melaena (i.e. black 'tarry' stool; ~65%) and shock (Chapter 4) if bleeding is severe. Occasionally fresh blood is passed rectally after large upper GI bleeds. Epigastric pain and tenderness suggest peptic ulceration. Stigmata of chronic liver disease (CLD), hepatosplenomegaly, mucocutaneous changes (e.g. hereditary haemorrhagic telangiectasia (HHT), Peutz–Jeghers syndrome) and bleeding disorders must be sought. Angiodysplasia is common in chronic renal failure (CRF). A history of retching or vomiting raises the possibility of a gastro-oesophageal tear (Mallory–Weiss syndrome). Anorexia, weight loss, lymph nodes and an epigastric mass indicate gastric carcinoma. An aortoenteric fistula may occur following aortic surgery. The drug history is essential (e.g. NSAIDs).

Investigation

- **Blood tests.** Haemoglobin levels do not fall immediately as haemodilution occurs over several hours. Microcytic, hypochromic anaemia suggests previous chronic bleeding. An elevated urea indicates upper rather than lower GI bleeding. Liver function tests and coagulation profile assess liver damage, synthetic function (e.g. albumin) and clotting dysfunction.
- **Diagnostic imaging.** Air beneath the diaphragm on chest or abdominal radiography indicates viscus perforation.

    Oesophagogastroduodenoscopy (OGD) or 'gastroscopy' is essential to establish the diagnosis, predict rebleeding risk (Table d) and treat bleeding lesions endoscopically.

    Angiography is indicated when OGD fails to locate a bleeding site (~20%) and bleeding continues.
- **Exploratory laparotomy** is required if life-threatening bleeding continues and other investigations are negative.

General management

- **Prophylactic therapies** to reduce the risk of upper GI bleeding include enteral nutrition, gastric acid suppression (e.g. omeprazole) and gastric mucosal coating (e.g. sucralphate).
- **General measures** include early involvement of the gastroenterologists and surgeons, supplemental oxygen and nasogastric tube drainage except in patients with varices.
- **Resuscitation.** Immediate plasma expanders are followed by blood transfusion (Chapter 5). Fresh frozen plasma and platelets are given as required (Chapter 41). Ongoing resuscitation is determined by haemodynamic parameters (Chapters 4, 5).

Peptic ulceration management

H_2-receptor antagonists (e.g. ranitidine) or proton pump inhibitors (PPIs, e.g. omeprazole) should be administered in upper GI bleeding when OGD confirms peptic ulceration or gastritis. Both drugs speed ulcer healing; however, PPIs reduce rebleeding more effectively. The value of tranexamic acid, an antifibrinolytic agent, and somatostatin or octreotide to reduce splanchnic blood flow is not established.

- **Endoscopy.** Thermal coagulation (e.g. bipolar electrocautery) and injection therapy (e.g. ethanol, adrenaline (epinephrine)) reduce ulcer rebleeding and the need for emergency surgery.
- **Surgery** is required for exsanguinating haemorrhage despite the associated mortality. A Billroth I gastrectomy is performed for bleeding gastric ulcers. Duodenal ulcers require oversewing and

vagotomy and pyloroplasty. Endoscopic therapy has reduced the need for surgery.
- **Arterial embolization** controls massive bleeding in 50% of high-risk surgical patients but may cause gastric necrosis.

Oesophageal varices management

Oesophageal varices require treatment of the underlying cause (e.g. cirrhosis) and associated liver failure.

- **Sclerotherapy** is the treatment of choice. Endoscopic injection of a sclerosant (e.g. alcohol, ethanolamine) thromboses varices and controls acute bleeding in >90%. Complications include ulceration and stricture formation.
- **Endoscopic variceal ligation (banding)** is equally effective.
- **Pharmacotherapy.** Vasopressin (or its longer-acting analogue terlipressin) lowers PrHT by causing splanchnic vasoconstriction. It controls variceal bleeding temporarily in 40–70% but may cause cardiac ischaemia. Somatostatin and octreotide are also effective. Beta-blockade reduces PrHT and is used as prophylaxis.
- **Balloon tamponade** (e.g. Sengstaken–Blakemore tube; Fig. c) is an effective temporizing measure to control massive bleeding.
- **Transjugular intrahepatic portal stent (TIPS)** is required if medical therapy fails. A self-expanding stent is positioned over a wire passed into the hepatic vein (via the transjugular route), then through the liver substance and into the portal vein, decompressing the portal system. Encephalopathy may ensue.
- **Surgery** including variceal ligation (e.g. transoesophageal stapling) or portocaval shunting is occasionally required.

Prognosis

Fortunately, upper GI bleeding stops spontaneously in 70% of cases, regardless of the cause. Mortality remains about 10%. Poor prognostic factors and risk factors for rebleeding include age >60 years, oesophageal varices (mortality ~40% with first bleed), gastric ulceration, coexisting disease and ongoing bleeding.

Lower gastrointestinal bleeding

Causes are listed in Table (e). Lower GI bleeding presents with either frank rectal bleeding or melaena (± shock). Abdominal examination may reveal a mass (e.g. neoplasia) or tenderness. A bruit suggests ischaemia. Angiodysplasia occurs in CRF, aortic stenosis and inherited vascular conditions (e.g. HHT). Investigation is as for upper GI bleeding but diagnostic imaging (in order of use) includes sigmoidoscopy, colonoscopy if OGD is negative, mesenteric arteriography (Fig. f), labelled red cell isotope scans or small bowel barium studies. Exploratory laparotomy may be necessary if profuse undiagnosed bleeding persists.

Management

Most bleeding stops spontaneously (~80%) but recurs in ~25%.
- **General management** is as for upper GI bleeding.
- **Specific measures** include: **endoscopy:** Colonoscopy with electrocoagulation or laser therapy can stop bleeding from polyps, angiodysplasia, telangiectasia and colorectal carcinomas. **Elective surgery** is frequently required for lower GI bleeding. Severe, persistent but undiagnosed bleeding due to presumed angiodysplasia may be treated with a right hemicolectomy, although this is an unsatisfactory compromise. **Arterial embolization** may be used for vascular mal-formations including angiodysplasia (Fig. f).

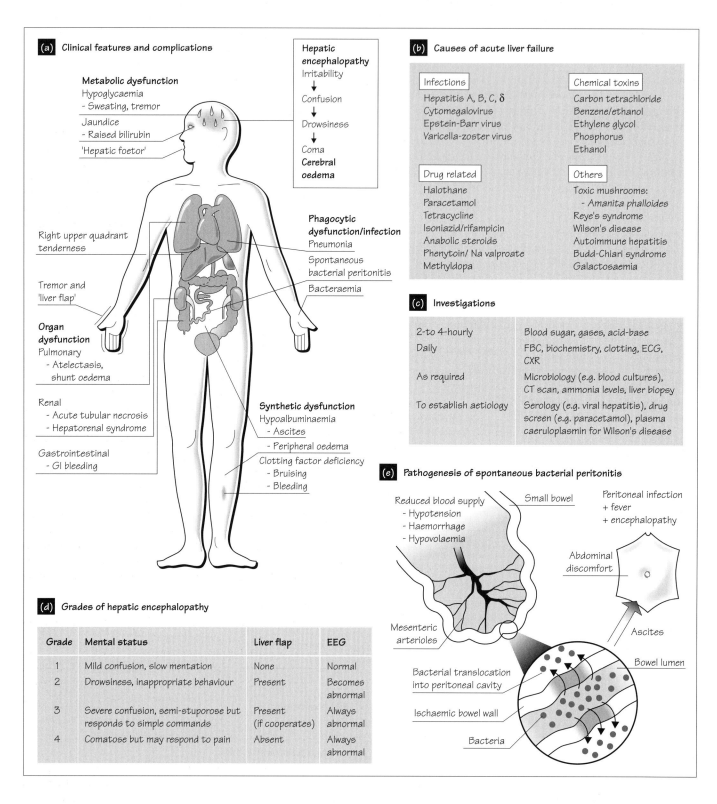

(a) Clinical features and complications

Metabolic dysfunction
Hypoglycaemia
- Sweating, tremor
Jaundice
- Raised bilirubin
'Hepatic foetor'

Hepatic encephalopathy
Irritability
↓
Confusion
↓
Drowsiness
↓
Coma
Cerebral oedema

Right upper quadrant tenderness

Tremor and 'liver flap'

Organ dysfunction
Pulmonary
- Atelectasis, shunt oedema

Renal
- Acute tubular necrosis
- Hepatorenal syndrome

Gastrointestinal
- GI bleeding

Phagocytic dysfunction/infection
Pneumonia
Spontaneous bacterial peritonitis
Bacteraemia

Synthetic dysfunction
Hypoalbuminaemia
- Ascites
- Peripheral oedema
Clotting factor deficiency
- Bruising
- Bleeding

(b) Causes of acute liver failure

Infections	Chemical toxins
Hepatitis A, B, C, δ	Carbon tetrachloride
Cytomegalovirus	Benzene/ethanol
Epstein-Barr virus	Ethylene glycol
Varicella-zoster virus	Phosphorus
	Ethanol

Drug related	Others
Halothane	Toxic mushrooms:
Paracetamol	- Amanita phalloides
Tetracycline	Reye's syndrome
Isoniazid/rifampicin	Wilson's disease
Anabolic steroids	Autoimmune hepatitis
Phenytoin/ Na valproate	Budd-Chiari syndrome
Methyldopa	Galactosaemia

(c) Investigations

2-to 4-hourly	Blood sugar, gases, acid-base
Daily	FBC, biochemistry, clotting, ECG, CXR
As required	Microbiology (e.g. blood cultures), CT scan, ammonia levels, liver biopsy
To establish aetiology	Serology (e.g. viral hepatitis), drug screen (e.g. paracetamol), plasma caeruloplasmin for Wilson's disease

(e) Pathogenesis of spontaneous bacterial peritonitis

Reduced blood supply
- Hypotension
- Haemorrhage
- Hypovolaemia

Small bowel

Peritoneal infection
+ fever
+ encephalopathy

Abdominal discomfort

Mesenteric arterioles

Ascites

Bacterial translocation into peritoneal cavity

Bowel lumen

Ischaemic bowel wall

Bacteria

(d) Grades of hepatic encephalopathy

Grade	Mental status	Liver flap	EEG
1	Mild confusion, slow mentation	None	Normal
2	Drowsiness, inappropriate behaviour	Present	Becomes abnormal
3	Severe confusion, semi-stuporose but responds to simple commands	Present (if cooperates)	Always abnormal
4	Comatose but may respond to pain	Absent	Always abnormal

- **Primary ALF (fulminant hepatic failure)** occurs in previously healthy people. It evolves over <4 weeks and is fatal in 75–90% of cases. Table (b) lists the causes. Viral hepatitis (~40–70%) and paracetamol toxicity (~40%) are most common. The main viral causes are hepatitis A (~30%) and hepatitis B (~25%). However, the risk of developing ALF from viral hepatitis is <1%. Paracetamol poisoning is discussed in Chapter 42.

- **Secondary ALF** is more frequent than primary ALF. It occurs when acute illness or stress causes decompensation in pre-existing chronic liver disease (CLD) including cirrhosis, chronic active hepatitis and metabolic disorders. In critical illness, ALF is due to ischaemic (e.g. shock, sepsis, hepatic vascular occlusion) or toxic liver damage (e.g. drugs, TPN).

Clinical features

Spider naevi, palmar erythema and ascites are features of pre-existing CLD. Biochemical and CNS dysfunction are hallmarks of ALF. Fig. (a) illustrates these features, which are due to:
- **Metabolic dysfunction.** Reduced hepatic gluconeogenesis and raised insulin levels cause hypoglycaemia in ~40%. Lactic acidosis occurs in ~50% due to poor lactate metabolism in late ALF.
  Liver function tests are raised (e.g. serum aminotransferase >2000 IU/L). Bilirubin increases and jaundice rapidly develops. The breath often has a sweetish smell, 'hepatic foetor', due to exhaled mercaptans. Ammonia levels are usually increased.
  Electrolyte disturbances (e.g. hyponatraemia, hypokalaemia) and secondary hyperaldosteronism are common.
- **Synthetic dysfunction** includes hypoalbuminaemia and clotting factor deficiencies. About 30% die with clotting disorders. GI bleeding causes ~20% of deaths (Chapter 34), and frequently precipitates shock and encephalopathy.
- **Reduced immunity.** Phagocytic dysfunction predisposes to infection but fever and leucocytosis only occur in ~30%. Death from bacteraemia occurs in ~15% and serious infections (e.g. pneumonia) develop in ~80%. Staphylococci, streptococci and Gram-negative rods are common organisms.
  Spontaneous bacterial peritonitis (SBP) is due to splanchnic hypoperfusion, which impairs bowel wall integrity, allowing bacterial translocation and peritoneal infection (Fig. e). Characteristic features are fever, abdominal discomfort and encephalopathy. Sudden onset of renal failure, weight gain or ascites also suggests SBP. Peritoneal fluid must be aspirated. Detection of bacteria confirms the diagnosis but a leucocyte count >500/mm^3, pH < 7.3 and raised lactate are also indications for treatment. Gram-negative rods (e.g. *E. coli*) are the commonest organism and blood cultures are positive in ~50%. Untreated SBP is fatal in 70–90%.
- **Organ dysfunction** progresses to multiple organ failure.
  Respiratory complications include pulmonary oedema due to hypoalbuminaemia and fluid overload. Pneumonia, atelectasis and pulmonary shunting due to failure of vasodilator clearance cause hypoxaemia.
  Renal failure affects ~50% due to hepatorenal syndrome (HRS) or ATN (Chapter 30). HRS causes oliguria insensitive to diuretics or fluids and has a high mortality.
  Cerebral oedema. Sudden cerebral herniation causes ~35% of deaths in ALF.
- **Hepatic encephalopathy (HpE)** is the most common fatal complication. It arises when toxin-laden portal blood bypasses the liver and is shunted into the systemic circulation.
  Precipitating factors include: (i) upper GI bleeding which increases gut protein and bacterial ammonia formation; (ii) intravascular volume depletion, which reduces hepatic perfusion (e.g. bleeding, diuretics); (iii) renal failure which impairs toxin/drug clearance; and (iv) infection.
  Clinical features. Early signs include altered mental status, irritability and confusion. Drowsiness and reduced consciousness develop over hours to weeks. Reversible causes must be excluded (e.g. hypoglycaemia, sedatives). Tremor, a liver 'flap' and sustained clonus can often be elicited.
  Diagnosis is clinical, supported by elevated ammonia levels and occasionally specific electroencephalogram (EEG) findings including high-amplitude δ and triphasic waves. However, most EEGs show non-specific diffuse slowing. HpE grades (Table d) are of limited value due to fluctuations in coma level.

Management

Essential investigations are listed in Table (c). Management is supportive apart from the use of N-acetylcysteine. In survivors, regeneration of liver may be associated with complete recovery.
- **General.** Early advice from or involvement of a specialist liver unit is *always* appropriate. Hypoglycaemia is prevented by glucose infusions (i.e. 10–20% dextrose). Detection and treatment of infection are essential but prophylactic antibiotics are ineffective. Antacids prevent stress ulceration but H$_2$ blockers can cause CNS side-effects due to impaired drug metabolism. Potassium supplements are often required.
  Nutrition. Avoid high protein loads and limit sodium intake. Branched-chain amino acids in TPN minimize HpE. Supplemental vitamin K, thiamine and folate are required.
- **Cardiorespiratory support** aims to maintain organ function. Appropriate resuscitation is paramount but excessive fluid therapy risks pulmonary oedema. Hypoxaemia (e.g. V/Q mismatch), inadequate ventilation (e.g. diaphragmatic splinting) or risk of aspiration may require early intubation and ventilation.
  Ascites, fluid retention (±hypokalaemia) are treated with potassium-sparing diuretics (e.g. spironolactone).
  Bleeding. Fresh frozen plasma (FFP) is required for invasive procedures and active bleeding but not prophylactically.
  Cerebral oedema. Hyperventilation and mannitol transiently reduce oedema but survival is not improved.
- **Encephalopathy** is prevented by avoiding sedation and correcting precipitating factors. Measures to reduce the nitrogenous load absorbed from the bowel include a low protein intake (<40 g/day), laxatives and non-absorbable antibiotics. If GI bleeding is suspected, lactulose reduces bowel transit time and prevents blood protein absorption. Convulsions are treated aggressively (Chapter 37).
- **Specific therapies** are limited.
  N-acetylcysteine benefits most patients but is essential in paracetamol-induced ALF (Chapter 42).
  Liver transplantation is a last resort with 1-year survivals between 50 and 75%. It has a limited but definite role in paracetamol-induced ALF but is less successful in alcohol-related ALF. Limited organ availability means that ~50% of candidates die awaiting a donor.

Prognosis

Overall survival rates for ALF are 20–30%. Mortality depends on cause (i.e. hepatitis A ~33–55%; paracetamol-induced ~47–65%; hepatitis B ~61–76%; and non-A, non-B hepatitis >85%), age (i.e. better if >10, <40 years old) and HpE grade. Other poor prognostic factors are bilirubin level (>18 mg/dL), metabolic acidosis (pH < 7.3), prothrombin time (>3.5) and organ failure (e.g. renal).

36 Acute pancreatitis

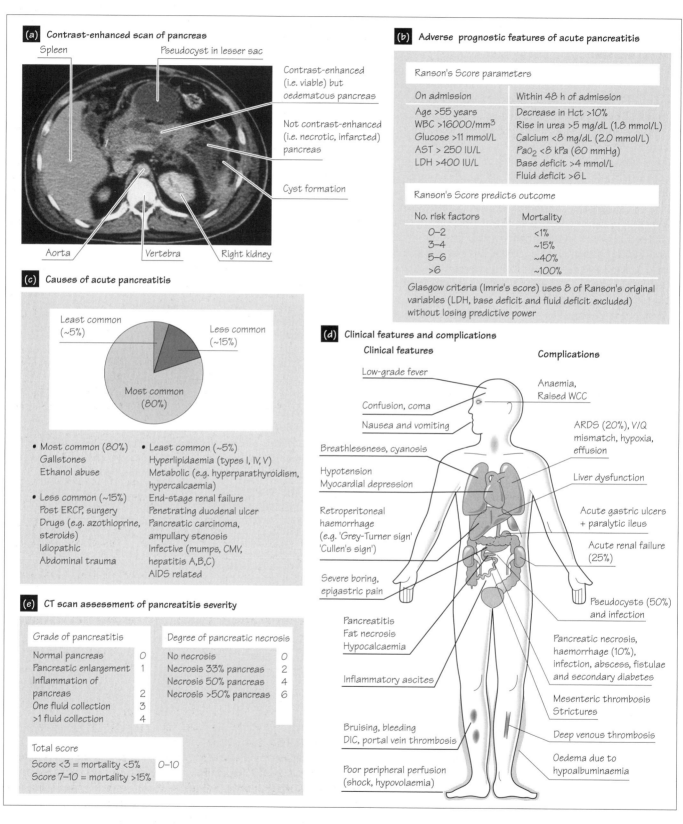

(a) Contrast-enhanced scan of pancreas

- Spleen
- Pseudocyst in lesser sac
- Contrast-enhanced (i.e. viable) but oedematous pancreas
- Not contrast-enhanced (i.e. necrotic, infarcted) pancreas
- Cyst formation
- Aorta
- Vertebra
- Right kidney

(b) Adverse prognostic features of acute pancreatitis

Ranson's Score parameters

On admission	Within 48 h of admission
Age >55 years	Decrease in Hct >10%
WBC >16000/mm^3	Rise in urea >5 mg/dL (1.8 mmol/L)
Glucose >11 mmol/L	Calcium <8 mg/dL (2.0 mmol/L)
AST > 250 IU/L	Pao$_2$ <8 kPa (60 mmHg)
LDH >400 IU/L	Base deficit >4 mmol/L
	Fluid deficit >6 L

Ranson's Score predicts outcome

No. risk factors	Mortality
0–2	<1%
3–4	~15%
5–6	~40%
>6	~100%

Glasgow criteria (Imrie's score) uses 8 of Ranson's original variables (LDH, base deficit and fluid deficit excluded) without losing predictive power

(c) Causes of acute pancreatitis

- Least common (~5%)
- Less common (~15%)
- Most common (80%)

- **Most common (80%)**
  Gallstones
  Ethanol abuse

- **Less common (~15%)**
  Post ERCP, surgery
  Drugs (e.g. azothioprine, steroids)
  Idiopathic
  Abdominal trauma

- **Least common (~5%)**
  Hyperlipidaemia (types I, IV, V)
  Metabolic (e.g. hyperparathyroidism, hypercalcaemia)
  End-stage renal failure
  Penetrating duodenal ulcer
  Pancreatic carcinoma, ampullary stenosis
  Infective (mumps, CMV, hepatitis A,B,C)
  AIDS related

(e) CT scan assessment of pancreatitis severity

Grade of pancreatitis		Degree of pancreatic necrosis	
Normal pancreas	0	No necrosis	0
Pancreatic enlargement	1	Necrosis 33% pancreas	2
Inflammation of pancreas	2	Necrosis 50% pancreas	4
One fluid collection	3	Necrosis >50% pancreas	6
>1 fluid collection	4		

Total score	
Score <3 = mortality <5%	0–10
Score 7–10 = mortality >15%	

(d) Clinical features and complications

Clinical features
- Low-grade fever
- Confusion, coma
- Nausea and vomiting
- Breathlessness, cyanosis
- Hypotension Myocardial depression
- Retroperitoneal haemorrhage (e.g. 'Grey-Turner sign' 'Cullen's sign')
- Severe boring, epigastric pain
- Pancreatitis Fat necrosis Hypocalcaemia
- Inflammatory ascites
- Bruising, bleeding DIC, portal vein thrombosis
- Poor peripheral perfusion (shock, hypovolaemia)

Complications
- Anaemia, Raised WCC
- ARDS (20%), V/Q mismatch, hypoxia, effusion
- Liver dysfunction
- Acute gastric ulcers + paralytic ileus
- Acute renal failure (25%)
- Pseudocysts (50%) and infection
- Pancreatic necrosis, haemorrhage (10%), infection, abscess, fistulae and secondary diabetes
- Mesenteric thrombosis Strictures
- Deep venous thrombosis
- Oedema due to hypoalbuminaemia

Acute pancreatitis may be clinically mild (75%) or severe (25%). Mild pancreatitis rarely requires ICU admission and resolves with analgesia and fluid therapy alone. In severe pancreatitis, prompt identification and ICU management of organ failures and local complications (e.g. necrosis, pseudocysts) improve outcome. However, mortality is still ~25%.

Aetiology

Causes. Gallstones and alcohol cause 80% of cases (Fig. c).
Pathogenesis. Ductal obstruction (e.g. gallstones) with biliary reflux into the pancreatic duct or cytotoxic injury (e.g. alcohol) initiates pancreatic autodigestion by the enzymes trypsin, lipase and elastase.
Histology. Acute pancreatitis is classified as **oedematous** (~75%) or **necrotizing** (~25%). Necrotic tissue is identified as failure of contrast enhancement on CT scanning (Fig. a).

Clinical features (Fig. d)

Pancreatitis presents with severe, persistent 'boring' epigastric and/or back pain. Nausea, vomiting and low-grade fever are common. Pain and fluid loss cause tachycardia, hypotension and shock. Acute lung injury may cause respiratory distress (Chapter 26). Peritonitis is unusual because the pancreas is retroperitoneal but epigastric tenderness and abdominal distension due to ileus are often present. Bruising in the loins (Grey–Turner's sign) and around the umbilicus (Cullen's sign) is a rare manifestation of retroperitoneal haemorrhage.

There are two clinical phases during severe pancreatitis.
1 *The early phase* (0–14 days) is due to inflammation (i.e. mediator release, SIRS) and large fluid shifts. It causes shock, ARDS, acute renal failure, coagulopathy, fat necrosis and hypocalcaemia.
2 *The late phase* is associated with local complications including pancreatic necrosis, infection (±abscess), pseudocyst, fistula, ascites, strictures, ileus, portal vein thrombosis and diabetes.

Investigation

• **Laboratory.** A raised WCC, uraemia, hypocalcaemia, hypoglycaemia and hypoalbuminaemia are common. Serum amylase levels 3–5 times normal are strongly suggestive of pancreatitis. However, amylase concentrations are raised in many abdominal emergencies but normal in ~30% of confirmed pancreatitis cases. Consequently, amylase levels have little prognostic value. Raised serum lipase is more specific but not widely available.
• **Radiological.** Abdominal X-rays may show localized ileus (e.g. 'sentinel loop', 'colon cut-off sign') or calcification in chronic pancreatitis. Abdominal USS detects gallstones, biliary duct dilation and pancreatic pseudocysts but pancreatic visualization is poor. CT scans best visualize the pancreas (e.g. oedema) and associated complications (e.g. necrosis) but only confirm the cause in ~25%.

Prognosis

Mortality is ~10% in sterile and ~35% in infected pancreatitis.
Early deaths (0–14 days) are due to SIRS and MOF.
Late deaths are usually due to infection, which develops in 40–60% of necrotizing pancreatitis. The risk of infection increases with the amount of necrosis and the time from onset.
Severity assessment. Several scoring systems assess severity and prognosis in pancreatitis (e.g. APACHE II). Of the specific scoring systems, Ranson's criteria are most commonly used (Table b). Other prognostic factors include: **(i) Cause (i.e. cytotoxic vs. gallstone):** death occurs early in alcohol-induced (i.e. inflammation-related) and later in gallstone-induced (i.e. sepsis-related) pancreatitis. Mortality is ~50% if the gallstone is not removed. Pancreatic haemorrhage carries the worst prognosis. **(ii) Histology (i.e. oedematous vs. necrotic):** necrosis is associated with increased mortality (Table e). **(iii) Pancreatic infection:** CT-guided fine needle aspiration reliably assesses the development of infection in necrotic tissue. **(iv) Multiorgan failure (MOF):** number of organ failures correlates with mortality.

Management

Uncomplicated, oedematous pancreatitis management includes:
1 *Fluid resuscitation and electrolyte replacement* to correct hypovolaemia due to 'third space' and GI (e.g. ileus, vomiting) losses. Inotropic support may be needed in severe pancreatitis.
2 *Nutrition.* Oral feeding is initially withheld (i.e to reduce pancreatic enzyme release) and nasogastric tube drainage initiated (although benefit has not been established). In uncomplicated pancreatitis, nutritional support is of limited value. However, in severe pancreatitis, early enteric feeding through a *nasojejunal tube* is well tolerated and reduces infectious complications. Parenteral nutrition is only justified if enteral feeding fails.
3 *Pain control* can be difficult. Theoretical concerns that morphine may evoke ampullary spasm are probably not justified but meperidine or pethidine analgesia may be preferred.
4 *Prophylactic antibiotics* are indicated in gallstone-induced pancreatitis because of the high incidence of biliary tract infection but not in other uncomplicated cases.
5 *Stress ulcer prophylaxis* (e.g. histamine blockers) reduces upper GI bleeding but pancreatitis is unaffected.
6 *Early gallstone extraction* reduces mortality, infective complications and severity of pancreatitis. ERCP is as successful as surgery if accomplished within 48 h.
7 *Specific medications* (e.g. anticholinergic, glucagon, octreotide) do not influence outcome in uncomplicated pancreatitis.

Severe necrotizing pancreatitis is treated as above, but since the development of infected necrosis substantially increases mortality, prevention and treatment of infection are essential.
1 *Antibiotic therapy* reduces infection and late mortality in necrotizing pancreatitis. High-dose cefuroxime or meropenem is started when necrosis is confirmed and continued for 2–4 weeks.
2 *Surgery.* Infected necrotizing pancreatitis is usually fatal without surgical debridement (necrosectomy). Endoscopic debridement techniques using irrigation are currently being assessed. In early sterile necrotizing pancreatitis, surgery does not reduce mortality but may be considered later in the disease for patients who remain systemically unwell (e.g. fever, weight loss).
3 *Somatostatin and octreotide* may improve outcome by reducing pancreatic secretions.

Complications and long-term sequelae

Complications of acute pancreatitis are illustrated in Fig. (d).
Pseudocysts are collections of pancreatic secretions and occur in ~50% of cases. Indications for drainage are pain, size >6 cm, gastric outlet obstruction and secondary infection or haemorrhage.
Chronic pancreatitis follows recurrent acute pancreatitis and causes chronic pain, pancreatic calcification and deficiency of endocrine and exocrine pancreatic function (e.g. malabsorption).

37 Altered mental state, coma and status epilepticus

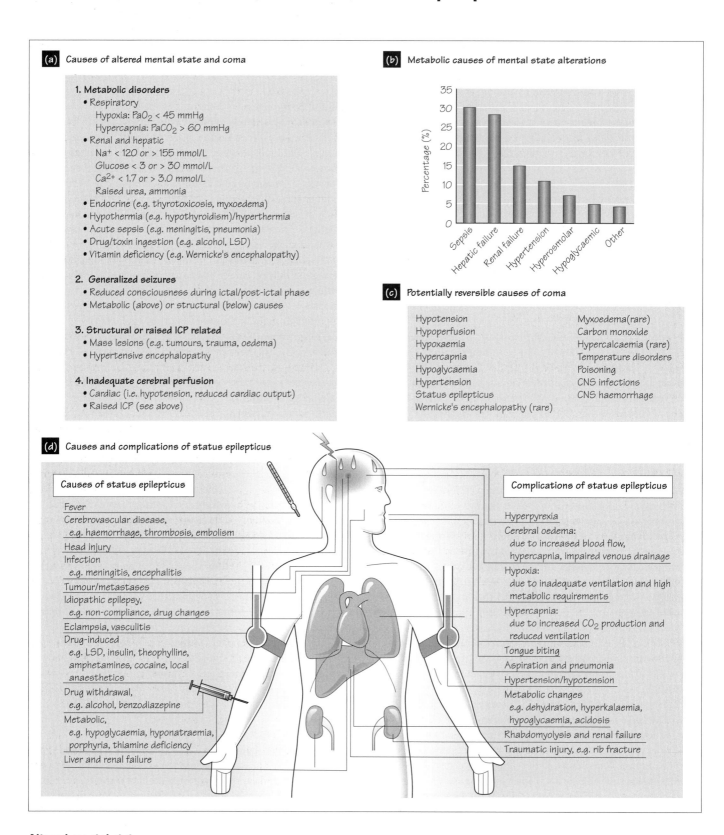

(a) Causes of altered mental state and coma

1. Metabolic disorders
- Respiratory
  Hypoxia: $PaO_2 < 45$ mmHg
  Hypercapnia: $PaCO_2 > 60$ mmHg
- Renal and hepatic
  $Na^+ < 120$ or > 155 mmol/L
  Glucose < 3 or > 30 mmol/L
  $Ca^{2+} < 1.7$ or 3.0 mmol/L
  Raised urea, ammonia
- Endocrine (e.g. thyrotoxicosis, myxoedema)
- Hypothermia (e.g. hypothyroidism)/hyperthermia
- Acute sepsis (e.g. meningitis, pneumonia)
- Drug/toxin ingestion (e.g. alcohol, LSD)
- Vitamin deficiency (e.g. Wernicke's encephalopathy)

2. Generalized seizures
- Reduced consciousness during ictal/post-ictal phase
- Metabolic (above) or structural (below) causes

3. Structural or raised ICP related
- Mass lesions (e.g. tumours, trauma, oedema)
- Hypertensive encephalopathy

4. Inadequate cerebral perfusion
- Cardiac (i.e. hypotension, reduced cardiac output)
- Raised ICP (see above)

(b) Metabolic causes of mental state alterations

Bar chart. Y-axis: Percentage (%), from 0 to 35. X-axis categories: Sepsis (~30), Hepatic failure (~28), Renal failure (~15), Hypertension (~11), Hyperosmolar (~7), Hypoglycaemic (~5), Other (~4)

(c) Potentially reversible causes of coma

Hypotension	Myxoedema (rare)
Hypoperfusion	Carbon monoxide
Hypoxaemia	Hypercalcaemia (rare)
Hypercapnia	Temperature disorders
Hypoglycaemia	Poisoning
Hypertension	CNS infections
Status epilepticus	CNS haemorrhage
Wernicke's encephalopathy (rare)	

(d) Causes and complications of status epilepticus

Causes of status epilepticus
- Fever
- Cerebrovascular disease,
  e.g. haemorrhage, thrombosis, embolism
- Head injury
- Infection
  e.g. meningitis, encephalitis
- Tumour/metastases
- Idiopathic epilepsy,
  e.g. non-compliance, drug changes
- Eclampsia, vasculitis
- Drug-induced
  e.g. LSD, insulin, theophylline,
  amphetamines, cocaine, local
  anaesthetics
- Drug withdrawal,
  e.g. alcohol, benzodiazepine
- Metabolic,
  e.g. hypoglycaemia, hyponatraemia,
  porphyria, thiamine deficiency
- Liver and renal failure

Complications of status epilepticus
- Hyperpyrexia
- Cerebral oedema:
  due to increased blood flow,
  hypercapnia, impaired venous drainage
- Hypoxia:
  due to inadequate ventilation and high
  metabolic requirements
- Hypercapnia:
  due to increased CO_2 production and
  reduced ventilation
- Tongue biting
- Aspiration and pneumonia
- Hypertension/hypotension
- Metabolic changes
  e.g. dehydration, hyperkalaemia,
  hypoglycaemia, acidosis
- Rhabdomyolysis and renal failure
- Traumatic injury, e.g. rib fracture

Altered mental state

Reduced consciousness is associated with disorientation, emotional lability, hallucinations and memory loss. It complicates many medical and surgical illnesses (Table a). Common precipitants are metabolic encephalopathy (Fig. b) and seizures. The elderly are most susceptible, and unless it is due to sedation, it is associated with increased mortality. Treatment must address the cause but occasionally cautious use of anxiolytics is required.

Coma

Definition. Coma is a state of unconsciousness from which the patient cannot be aroused. It is often defined as a Glasgow Coma Score (GCS; Chapter 45) of ≤8. Coma may be preceded by altered mental state or progressive loss of consciousness. The extent of neurological impairment depends on age, mental and cardiovascular status, underlying disease and rate of progression.

Pathophysiological causes include metabolic/toxic encephalopathy, generalized seizures, cerebral compression due to structural lesions (e.g. CVA) or raised intracranial pressure (ICP) and inadequate cerebral perfusion (Table a).

Assessment

History often determines the cause: trauma, hypothermia, drug/alcohol abuse and previous illness (e.g. diabetes, liver failure, atrial fibrillation (i.e. embolic stroke), etc.). Sudden onset suggests a seizure or vascular event, whereas a slower onset suggests a metabolic cause, tumour or extradural haematoma.

Examination. Vital signs aid differential diagnosis (Table a). Head injury must be excluded and, if suspicious, immobilize the cervical spine. Examine for meningism, liver or renal disease, and venepuncture marks (i.e. illicit drug use). The key features of neurological examination (mnemonic: SPERM) are:

(i) *States of consciousness* including alert, lethargic (i.e. responds to simple commands), stuporous (i.e. aroused by vigorous stimulation/pain) or comatose (i.e. unrousable). Record the GCS.

(ii) *Pupillary responses* which are controlled in the midbrain and if normal suggest coma is due to a metabolic cause or a structural lesion above the midbrain. Bilateral unreactive or pinpoint pupils suggest brainstem pathology. Many drugs affect pupillary response (e.g. morphine causes pinpoint pupils).

(iii) *Eye movement* which requires intact pontomedullary–midbrain connections. Normally, if the head turns, the gaze will initially remain fixed in the original direction (oculocephalic testing) or, if iced water is injected into the ear at the tympanic membrane, eye nystagmus and deviation towards the stimulated side occurs (oculovestibular testing). If these tests produce no change in the central eye position, the pons is non-functional.

(iv) *Respiratory pattern.* Tachypnoea is non-specific but may indicate acidosis, hypoxaemia or altered respiratory control. Ataxic breathing is a marker of severe brainstem dysfunction.

(v) *Motor function.* The best response is noted (e.g. spontaneously moves all limbs, no response to pain). Pontine compression often causes decerebrate (i.e. extensor) posturing, whereas lesions above the pons cause decorticate (i.e. flexor) posturing.

Full neurological examination may localize focal signs and differentiate between structural and metabolic causes. Incontinence and tongue lacerations indicate seizure.

Management

Investigations depend on the cause but include biochemistry, toxicology (with blood alcohol level), blood gases, carboxyhaemoglobin level, CT scan, EEG and lumbar puncture in the absence of raised ICP.

Treatment. After the airway has been secured common reversible causes of coma must be identified (Table c) and corrected. Intuba-

tion may be required if GCS is <10 to protect the airway and to facilitate investigation (e.g. CT scan). Hypoglycaemia and electrolyte imbalance are corrected. Thiamine is administered if alcohol abuse is suspected. The specific antagonists naloxone and flumazenil temporarily reverse narcotic- and benzodiazepine-induced coma, respectively (Chapter 13). Subsequent management including anticoagulants, anticonvulsants and ICP reduction depend on differentiation between neurological and medical causes of coma (Chapters 38, 45, 49).

Prognosis and monitoring coma. The GCS is a prognostic, reproducible method of assessing patient responsiveness and is described in Chapter 45. Prognosis can also be judged from posture and pupillary and oculovestibular reflexes, but only after drug, metabolic, cranial nerve and tympanic membrane defects have been excluded (Chapters 17, 45). Prognosis deteriorates with duration of coma. Patients with postanoxic coma (i.e. cardiac arrest) for >3 days rarely survive without severe disability. Poor prognosis is associated with decerebrate posturing and rigidity for >24h in non-trauma and >2 weeks in trauma patients; absent pupillary reflexes for >24h in postanoxic brain injury or >3 days for other patients; and absent oculovestibular reflexes for >24h.

Status epilepticus

Status epilepticus (SEp) is defined as prolonged seizure (>30 min duration) or recurrent, closely packed seizures without intervening return to consciousness. Prolonged seizures irreversibly damage brain tissue due to hypoxia, hypotension, cerebral oedema and direct neuronal injury. Damage is proportional to seizure duration, with mortality rates of 15–30%.

Causes (Fig. d). Patients with epilepsy and metabolic disturbances have a good prognosis, whereas those with global hypoxia, structural damage or infective lesions have a poor prognosis.

Clinical features and complications (Fig. d). Severe lactic acidosis (i.e. pH < 7.0), metabolic imbalance, high fever, cerebral oedema and raised ICP accompany SEp.

Investigations include routine blood tests and toxicology. Anticonvulsant levels are checked and corrected in known epileptics. In patients with new-onset seizures, CT imaging identifies structural lesions and EEG differentiates primary and secondary (focal) generalized seizures. In undiagnosed coma the EEG occasionally reveals unexpected SEp.

Management

Primary considerations are airway protection to prevent aspiration (i.e. lateral decubitus position, endotracheal intubation), supplemental oxygen and circulatory support. Correct pyrexia, hypoglycaemia and electrolyte disturbances. Hypotonic fluids that increase cerebral oedema should be avoided. In severe SEp, continuous EEG monitoring is indicated.

- **Anticonvulsants.** Rapid control of seizure activity is achieved with intravenous or rectal benzodiazepines (e.g. diazepam, lorazepam). Lasting seizure control is usually achieved with phenytoin. In resistant SEp, alternative therapies include sodium valproate, vigabatrin, barbiturates (e.g. phenobarbitone) and intravenous anaesthetic agents (e.g. propofol and thiopentone).
- **Other therapies** include hyperventilation and osmotic diuretics for cerebral oedema; steroids for tumours and arteritis; thiamine supplements for alcoholics; and surgery for space-occupying lesions (e.g. haemorrhage).

(a) Clinical features of stroke

Feature	Thrombotic	Embolic	Haemorrhagic
Time course	Slow, stuttering onset	Sudden, maximal defect	Abrupt, rapid onset
Location	Cortical infarcts	Cortical infarcts	Internal capsule, cortical, basal ganglia
Preceding history	TIA ± amaurosis fugax Retinal artery occlusion	Recent MI Arrhythmias (e.g. AF)	Anticoagulation Recent thrombolysis
Predisposing factors	DM, smoking, HT, hyperlipidaemia, heart disease	Endocarditis, ASD + PE, LV aneurysm and thrombus, air embolism, AF	HT, vascular malformation, herald bleeds and headache, cardiac catheterization
Treatment	Endarterectomy Aspirin (± thrombolysis?)	Aspirin anticoagulation	Surgical evacuation Correct coagulopathy

(b) Haemorrhagic stroke on CT scan showing 'bright white' blood

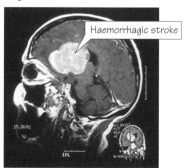

Haemorrhagic stroke

(c) Dilated left pupil and carotid angiogram showing leaking berry aneurysm

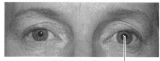

Dilated left pupil

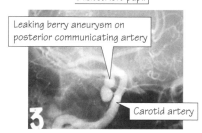

Leaking berry aneurysm on posterior communicating artery

Carotid artery

A 44-year-old woman presents with severe headache and dilated left pupil due to the pressure of a posterior communicating aneurysm on the pupillary parasympathetic 'constrictor' fibres lying on the surface of the left third cranial nerve

Cerebrovascular accident (CVA)

CVAs are focal neurological deficits of abrupt, non-traumatic origin lasting >24h. Patients are usually treated on medical wards. However, CVA can occur during critical illness, presenting as agitation, confusion or seizures. Thromboembolic (TE) events cause ~80% and intracerebral haemorrhage (ICH) ~20% of CVAs. Table (a) summarizes clinical features. **(i) Thrombotic CVA** follows atherothrombosis, vasculitis or coagulopathy. In hypertension (HT), small internal capsule infarcts cause large functional deficits. CT scans reveal hypodense areas. Haemorrhage occurs in large infarcts. **(ii) Embolic CVAs** are less common. Arterial procedures, arrhythmias, endocarditis and surgery increase the risk. **(iii) Haemorrhagic CVAs** occur in the basal ganglia (~50%) or pons (~5%) due to HT and in the cortex or cerebellum (~45%) due to arteriovenous malformations (AVMs). Other risk factors are drug abuse (e.g. cocaine), anticoagulation and thrombolysis. CT scans confirm the diagnosis (Fig. b). Mortality is ~50%.
Clinical features: Basal ganglia and cortical CVAs often cause hemiplegia. Quadraparesis, pinpoint pupils, coma and midposition eyes indicate pons lesions. Cerebellar lesions cause ataxia, nausea and vomiting. **Management** includes treatment of hypoxia, arrhythmias and associated seizures. Rapid BP reduction may be harmful (Chapter 22). In TE strokes aspirin improves outcome. Thrombolysis increases mortality due to ICH, although survivors have less neurological impairment. Anticoagulation is contraindicated in haemorrhagic infarcts, HT or large strokes. Patients at risk of emboli are anticoagulated after 48h, if repeat CT scanning excludes haemorrhage. Surgical evacuation improves outcome in cerebellar haemorrhage. Prophylactic measures prevent DVT (~30%), peptic ulceration, pressure sores and aspiration.

Subarachnoid haemorrhage (SAH)

SAH is spontaneous bleeding from intracranial aneurysms (~85%; Fig. c) or AVM (~15%). Risk factors include family history of SAH, connective tissue disease, polycystic disease and HT.
Clinical features. SAH presents as sudden headache, sometimes described as a 'blow to the back of the neck', with nausea, vomit-

ing, confusion or coma. The headache is not always severe. Neck stiffness, subhyaloid haemorrhage (~25%) and focal neurological signs due to vasospasm or mass effect develop later. Complications include arrhythmias, pulmonary oedema and hydrocephalus. Grading systems use symptom severity, GCS and motor deficit.
Investigation. CT imaging (± lumbar puncture) detects >95% of SAH within 24h. Angiography (Fig. c) locates the aneurysm (~80% anterior cerebral circulation).
Treatment requires resuscitation, analgesia and anticonvulsants. Nimodipine, a calcium channel blocker, prevents cerebral artery vasospasm. Surgery clips whereas radiological endovascular procedures thrombose the aneurysm.
Prognosis. Initial mortality is ~40%, and ~25% have recurrent bleeds if early surgical repair is not feasible. Severe neurological deficits affect ~30% of survivors.

Extradural haematoma is due to middle meningeal artery rupture after head injury. A lucid period precedes rapid GCS deterioration. Prognosis is good following early surgical drainage. **Subdural haematomas** are associated with severe traumatic brain injury, low GCS and poor prognosis.

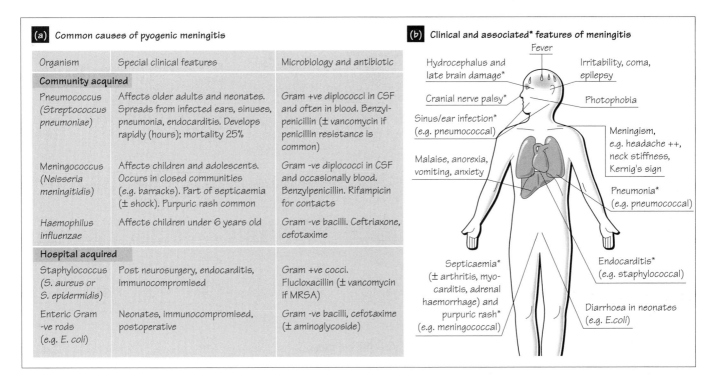

(a) Common causes of pyogenic meningitis

Organism	Special clinical features	Microbiology and antibiotic
Community acquired		
Pneumococcus (*Streptococcus pneumoniae*)	Affects older adults and neonates. Spreads from infected ears, sinuses, pneumonia, endocarditis. Develops rapidly (hours); mortality 25%	Gram +ve diplococci in CSF and often in blood. Benzyl-penicillin (± vancomycin if penicillin resistance is common)
Meningococcus (*Neisseria meningitidis*)	Affects children and adolescents. Occurs in closed communities (e.g. barracks). Part of septicaemia (± shock). Purpuric rash common	Gram -ve diplococci in CSF and occasionally blood. Benzylpenicillin. Rifampicin for contacts
Haemophilus influenzae	Affects children under 6 years old	Gram -ve bacilli. Ceftriaxone, cefotaxime
Hospital acquired		
Staphylococcus (*S. aureus* or *S. epidermidis*)	Post neurosurgery, endocarditis, immunocompromised	Gram +ve cocci. Flucloxacillin (± vancomycin if MRSA)
Enteric Gram -ve rods (e.g. *E. coli*)	Neonates, immunocompromised, postoperative	Gram -ve bacilli, cefotaxime (± aminoglycoside)

(b) Clinical and associated* features of meningitis

Fever
Hydrocephalus and late brain damage*
Irritability, coma, epilepsy
Cranial nerve palsy*
Photophobia
Sinus/ear infection* (e.g. pneumococcal)
Meningism, e.g. headache ++, neck stiffness, Kernig's sign
Malaise, anorexia, vomiting, anxiety
Pneumonia* (e.g. pneumococcal)
Septicaemia* (± arthritis, myo-carditis, adrenal haemorrhage) and purpuric rash* (e.g. meningococcal)
Endocarditis* (e.g. staphylococcal)
Diarrhoea in neonates (e.g. *E.coli*)

Meningitis

Meningitis is a life-threatening but treatable infection if rapidly recognized. It is suspected in any patient with mental state changes and fever. Signs of meningeal irritation are not always present.

Causes. Table (a) lists the common bacterial causes. Viruses (e.g. coxsackie, mumps), *Mycobacterium tuberculosis* (TB) and leptospirosis (Weil's disease) present less acutely. *Listeria monocytogenes* and *Cryptococcus neoformans* meningitis mainly affect immunocompromised patients (e.g. AIDS).

Clinical features (Fig. b) include infection (e.g. septicaemia), meningism and raised ICP. Precipitating causes must be excluded (e.g. pneumococcal meningitis is often secondary to chest, ear or sinus infections). Chronic TB meningitis is easily missed. SAH, malignancy and abscess may present with meningism. **Complications** include seizures (~30%), cerebral oedema, obstructive hydrocephalus and inappropriate antidiuretic hormone syndrome.

Investigation. In the absence of papilloedema or focal neurological deficits, lumbar puncture may be performed safely without a CT scan. Cerebrospinal fluid (CSF) in bacterial infections reveals raised polymorphs (>500/mm³), increased protein (0.5–3 g/L), low CSF:blood sugar ratio (CSF:BS < 40%) and bacteria on stain or culture. Blood cultures may also be positive. In viral meningitis CSF demonstrates raised lymphocytes (<500/mm³) and protein (0.5–1 g/L), but normal CSF:BS ratio (~60%). Viral culture and immunology of CSF, throat swabs or faeces are diagnostic. In TB meningitis CSF shows raised lymphocytes (<500/mm³) and protein (1–5 g/L) and a low CSF:BS ratio (<40%). Acid-fast bacilli on staining or culture confirm the diagnosis. India ink stains detect *Cryptococcus*.

Treatment (Table a). Benzylpenicillin is effective against most community-acquired pneumococcal or meningococcal meningitis.

H. influenzae is treated with cefotaxime or ceftriaxone. If an organism is not isolated, empirical cefotaxime (±penicillin) is started and cultures awaited. Aminoglycosides and antistaphylococcal cover are required in hospital-acquired meningitis. TB meningitis is treated with standard quadruple therapy. Steroids improve outcome and reduce complications in bacterial and tuberculous meningitis. Rifampicin is given to close contacts of meningococcal and *H. influenzae* meningitis.

Encephalitis

Encephalitis is an acute, usually viral, brain infection (e.g. herpes simplex). It is a rare complication of common viral diseases like chickenpox and mumps. Immunocompromised patients are at greatest risk. Initial features include drowsiness, irritability, fever, meningism and occasionally focal neurological signs. Severe cases progress to seizures, coma and death. CSF reveals lymphocytosis and raised protein. Viral serology may identify the cause. Management is supportive but aciclovir treats herpes simplex and ganciclovir, CMV infections. Prognosis varies but mortality is high with some infections (e.g. Japanese B virus).

Other neurological infections

These occur in countries with poor immunization programmes. **Tetanus** is a toxin-mediated disease caused by *Clostridium tetani* infection of necrotic wounds. Generalized muscle rigidity, spasms and respiratory failure require heavy sedation, paralysis and mechanical ventilation. Severe cardiovascular instability is controlled with magnesium infusions. Antibiotics, surgical debridement and immune globulin treat the infection and toxin. **Poliomyelitis, botulism and rabies** also cause paralytic neurological infections.

40 Neuromuscular conditions

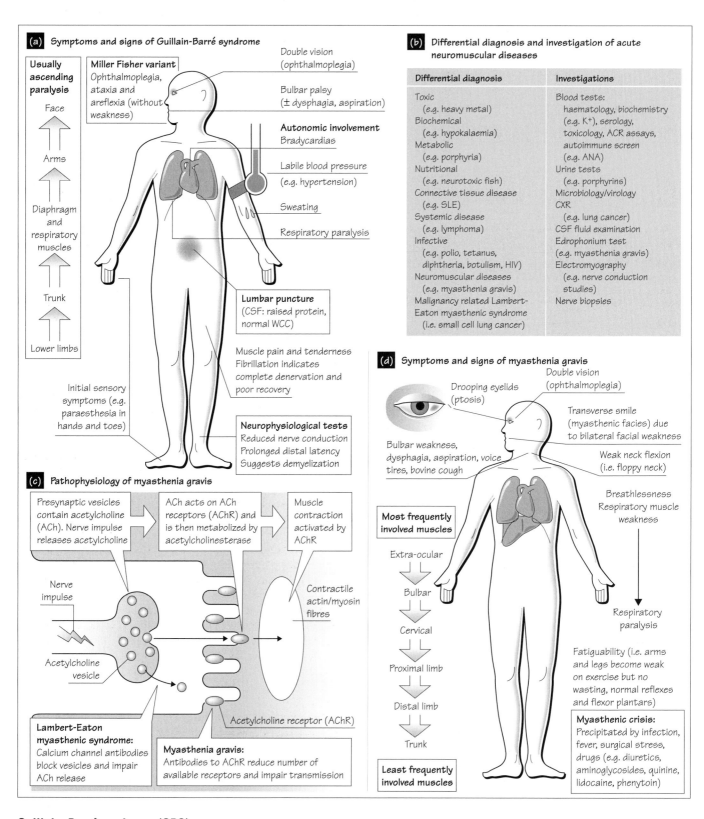

(a) Symptoms and signs of Guillain-Barré syndrome

Usually ascending paralysis
Face → Arms → Diaphragm and respiratory muscles → Trunk → Lower limbs

Miller Fisher variant
Ophthalmoplegia, ataxia and areflexia (without weakness)

Double vision (ophthalmoplegia)

Bulbar palsy (± dysphagia, aspiration)

Autonomic involvement
Bradycardias

Labile blood pressure (e.g. hypertension)

Sweating

Respiratory paralysis

Lumbar puncture (CSF: raised protein, normal WCC)

Muscle pain and tenderness
Fibrillation indicates complete denervation and poor recovery

Initial sensory symptoms (e.g. paraesthesia in hands and toes)

Neurophysiological tests
Reduced nerve conduction
Prolonged distal latency
Suggests demyelization

(b) Differential diagnosis and investigation of acute neuromuscular diseases

Differential diagnosis	Investigations
Toxic (e.g. heavy metal)	Blood tests: haematology, biochemistry (e.g. K+), serology, toxicology, ACR assays, autoimmune screen (e.g. ANA)
Biochemical (e.g. hypokalaemia)	
Metabolic (e.g. porphyria)	
Nutritional (e.g. neurotoxic fish)	Urine tests (e.g. porphyrins)
Connective tissue disease (e.g. SLE)	Microbiology/virology
Systemic disease (e.g. lymphoma)	CXR (e.g. lung cancer)
Infective (e.g. polio, tetanus, diphtheria, botulism, HIV)	CSF fluid examination
	Edrophonium test (e.g. myasthenia gravis)
Neuromuscular diseases (e.g. myasthenia gravis)	Electromyography (e.g. nerve conduction studies)
Malignancy related Lambert-Eaton myasthenic syndrome (i.e. small cell lung cancer)	Nerve biopsies

(c) Pathophysiology of myasthenia gravis

Presynaptic vesicles contain acetylcholine (ACh). Nerve impulse releases acetylcholine

ACh acts on ACh receptors (AChR) and is then metabolized by acetylcholinesterase

Muscle contraction activated by AChR

Nerve impulse

Contractile actin/myosin fibres

Acetylcholine vesicle

Acetylcholine receptor (AChR)

Lambert-Eaton myasthenic syndrome:
Calcium channel antibodies block vesicles and impair ACh release

Myasthenia gravis:
Antibodies to AChR reduce number of available receptors and impair transmission

(d) Symptoms and signs of myasthenia gravis

Drooping eyelids (ptosis)

Double vision (ophthalmoplegia)

Transverse smile (myasthenic facies) due to bilateral facial weakness

Bulbar weakness, dysphagia, aspiration, voice tires, bovine cough

Weak neck flexion (i.e. floppy neck)

Breathlessness
Respiratory muscle weakness

Most frequently involved muscles

Extra-ocular → Bulbar → Cervical → Proximal limb → Distal limb → Trunk

Least frequently involved muscles

Respiratory paralysis

Fatiguability (i.e. arms and legs become weak on exercise but no wasting, normal reflexes and flexor plantars)

Myasthenic crisis:
Precipitated by infection, fever, surgical stress, drugs (e.g. diuretics, aminoglycosides, quinine, lidocaine, phenytoin)

Guillain–Barré syndrome (GBS)

GBS is the commonest cause of acute generalized flaccid paralysis, affecting ~1.5/10^5 population each year.

Pathophysiology is a postinfective, acute, inflammatory, demyelinating polyradiculoneuropathy. A short-lived flu-like illness precedes ~70% of cases. It also follows Epstein–Barr virus, CMV,

HIV, hepatitis or *Campylobacter jejuni* infections. The probable mechanism is cross-reactivity of the immune response to the infecting organism with peripheral nerves. GBS is differentiated from other acute neuropathies (Table b) and chronic inflammatory demyelinating polyneuropathy (CIDP) which is usually idiopathic but can occur in HIV infection.

Clinical features (Fig. a). Initial symptoms are often sensory with distal paraesthesia. Weakness, areflexia and paralysis follow, usually ascending from the lower limbs to the face. In severe cases, respiratory, bulbar (e.g. extraocular muscle paralysis) and autonomic involvement (e.g. bradycardia) occur. **Clinical variants** include **Miller–Fisher syndrome** with ophthalmoplegia, ataxia and areflexia, and the **axonal form** which has a rapid onset and poor prognosis and is associated with anti-GM_1 ganglioside antibodies and *C. jejuni* infection.

Prognosis. Rapid progression can cause flaccid quadriparesis and respiratory paralysis within 24–72 h. Overall, ~30% require mechanical ventilation (MV) for between a few days to >1 year. Maximum neurological deficit occurs at ~14–21 days, followed by gradual recovery over weeks or months. Mortality is <10% but ~10% of survivors have residual neurological deficits. Prognosis is worse in the elderly and those with rapid onset and axonal damage.

Investigations (Table b) must exclude other causes of progressive weakness (e.g. hypokalaemia, tetanus). **Electrophysiology** detects reduced nerve conduction velocity and prolonged distal latency suggesting demyelination. **CSF examination** finds raised protein (>0.5 g/L) with normal white cell counts.

Management. Respiratory and autonomic function (e.g. BP) are monitored. **Respiratory reserve** is determined by 4-hourly vital capacity (VC) measurements. Respiratory distress and blood gas deterioration are late features of respiratory failure. Elective intubation is indicated if VC approaches 15 mL/kg (~1 L) or pharyngeal paralysis impairs secretion clearance. Respiratory function usually recovers within 2–3 weeks but a tracheostomy is required if paralysis persists. Chest physiotherapy and microbiological monitoring reduce respiratory infections. **Autonomic dysfunction** is minimized with fluid resuscitation and sedation. Profound bradycardia may require temporary pacemaker insertion.

General measures include skin care, nutrition, analgesia (e.g. neuropathic pain), thromboembolic prophylaxis and physiotherapy to prevent joint contractures. **Specific measures** include high-dose intravenous immunoglobulin and plasma exchange. Both speed recovery if used early. Steroids are of no benefit except for radicular (root) pain and CIDP.

Myasthenia gravis (MG)

MG is an autoimmune disorder characterized by skeletal muscle fatiguability and weakness. Antibodies to nicotinic, postsynaptic, acetylcholine receptors (AChRs) are detected in ~90%. AChR loss reduces transmission across the neuromuscular junction (Fig. c). It affects $5/10^5$ population, usually women aged 20–30 years old. Men are affected later (>50 years old). Thymus gland abnormalities occur in ~75%, usually thymic hyperplasia in young females and benign thymomas (~10%) in elderly males. MG is associated with autoimmune disorders (e.g. thyroid disease ~10%), genetic factors (i.e. HLA-linked), drug therapy (e.g. penicillamine) and bone marrow transplant rejection.

Clinical features (Fig. d). MG usually develops insidiously over weeks. Typically muscle weakness increases with repetitive use and recovers with rest. Extraocular muscles are most frequently involved, trunk muscles least (Fig. d). Ptosis and diplopia are the commonest presenting features. MG is confined to the extraocular muscles in ~20%. Bulbar muscle involvement causes dysphagia, aspiration and a snarling smile (myasthenic facies). **Myasthenic crisis** describes a life-threatening deterioration of MG precipitated by infection, fever, surgical stress or drugs (e.g. aminoglycosides). Rapid respiratory failure requires intubation and MV.

Investigations include blood for AChR antibodies. CXR and CT scans exclude thymoma. **Electromyography** shows a rapid decline in muscle action potentials on repetitive stimulation. **The edrophonium (Tensilon) test** is diagnostic. Edrophonium prevents breakdown of acetylcholine by acetylcholinesterase. Increased acetylcholine temporarily restores neuromuscular transmission, abolishing weakness, ptosis and diplopia. However, muscarinic AChR stimulation may cause autonomic side-effects (e.g. sweating, bradycardia) requiring treatment with atropine. Initially a test dose of edrophonium (e.g. 2 mg) is injected and, if muscarinic side-effects are not excessive, a further 8 mg is given. Improved strength within 1 min that lasts for several minutes supports the diagnosis of MG. Facilities for intubation must be available because excess acetylcholine inhibits neuromuscular transmission and may precipitate a **cholinergic crisis** (e.g. apnoea, paralysis, bulbar palsy, excessive secretions, colic).

Management. Monitor respiratory function in patients with dyspnoea or difficulty swallowing. Consider elective intubation if the VC falls below 15 mL/kg (~1 L), or if secretion clearance is inadequate. MV is required in ~10%. Check swallowing in dysphagic patients and start thromboembolic prophylaxis.

Specific treatment includes the following. **(i) Anticholinesterase drugs** (e.g. pyridostigmine) which provide symptomatic relief. The dose is slowly increased to achieve optimum benefit. However, excessive doses in an attempt to abolish all weakness may result in cholinergic crisis. Anticholinergics may be required to control muscarinic side-effects (e.g. salivation, colic, diarrhoea). **(ii) Immunosuppressive therapy.** Steroids may benefit patients with ocular symptoms alone or suboptimal responses to anticholinesterases. Initial deterioration is followed by improvement after several weeks. Azathioprine is required for severe MG. **(iii) Plasma exchange** produces short-lived (~4 weeks) but marked improvements during myasthenic crisis or ventilator weaning. **(iv) Thymectomy** improves ~80% of MG; onset of remission is more rapid and mortality lower than with medical therapy alone.

Other disorders

Many neuromuscular diseases (e.g. polio) require critical care support, most frequently following respiratory failure or surgical interventions.

Critical illness polyneuropathy occurs after sepsis, MOF or high-dose steroids, particularly if combined with prolonged paralysis. Axonal degeneration of the motor (± sensory) peripheral nerves leads to weakness, wasting, weaning failure and loss of reflexes. Nerve conduction studies confirm axonal loss. Treatment is symptomatic, and recovery may take many months.

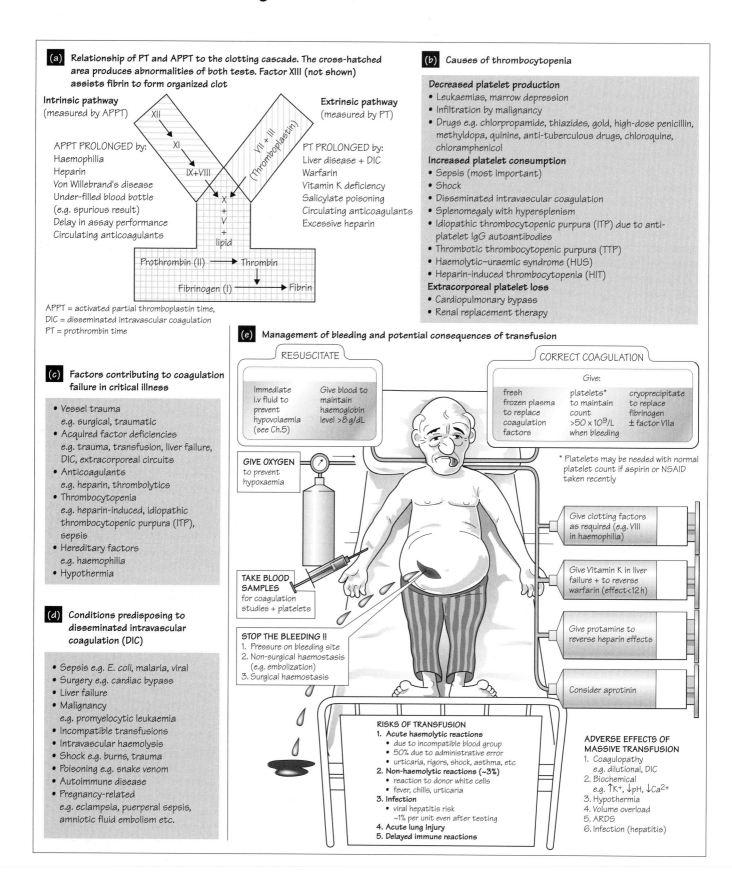

(a) Relationship of PT and APPT to the clotting cascade. The cross-hatched area produces abnormalities of both tests. Factor XIII (not shown) assists fibrin to form organized clot

Intrinsic pathway
(measured by APPT)

Extrinsic pathway
(measured by PT)

XII

XI

IX+VIII

VII + III
(Thromboplastin)

APPT PROLONGED by:
Haemophilia
Heparin
Von Willebrand's disease
Under-filled blood bottle
(e.g. spurious result)
Delay in assay performance
Circulating anticoagulants

PT PROLONGED by:
Liver disease + DIC
Warfarin
Vitamin K deficiency
Salicylate poisoning
Circulating anticoagulants
Excessive heparin

X
+
V
+
lipid

Prothrombin (II) → Thrombin

Fibrinogen (I) → Fibrin

APPT = activated partial thromboplastin time,
DIC = disseminated intravascular coagulation
PT = prothrombin time

(b) Causes of thrombocytopenia

Decreased platelet production
- Leukaemias, marrow depression
- Infiltration by malignancy
- Drugs e.g. chlorpropamide, thiazides, gold, high-dose penicillin, methyldopa, quinine, anti-tuberculous drugs, chloroquine, chloramphenicol

Increased platelet consumption
- Sepsis (most important)
- Shock
- Disseminated intravascular coagulation
- Splenomegaly with hypersplenism
- Idiopathic thrombocytopenic purpura (ITP) due to anti-platelet IgG autoantibodies
- Thrombotic thrombocytopenic purpura (TTP)
- Haemolytic–uraemic syndrome (HUS)
- Heparin-induced thrombocytopenia (HIT)

Extracorporeal platelet loss
- Cardiopulmonary bypass
- Renal replacement therapy

(c) Factors contributing to coagulation failure in critical illness

- Vessel trauma
  e.g. surgical, traumatic
- Acquired factor deficiencies
  e.g. trauma, transfusion, liver failure, DIC, extracorporeal circuits
- Anticoagulants
  e.g. heparin, thrombolytics
- Thrombocytopenia
  e.g. heparin-induced, idiopathic thrombocytopenic purpura (ITP), sepsis
- Hereditary factors
  e.g. haemophilia
- Hypothermia

(d) Conditions predisposing to disseminated intravascular coagulation (DIC)

- Sepsis e.g. E. coli, malaria, viral
- Surgery e.g. cardiac bypass
- Liver failure
- Malignancy
  e.g. promyelocytic leukaemia
- Incompatible transfusions
- Intravascular haemolysis
- Shock e.g. burns, trauma
- Poisoning e.g. snake venom
- Autoimmune disease
- Pregnancy-related
  e.g. eclampsia, puerperal sepsis, amniotic fluid embolism etc.

(e) Management of bleeding and potential consequences of transfusion

RESUSCITATE

Immediate i.v fluid to prevent hypovolaemia (see Ch.5)

Give blood to maintain haemoglobin level >8 g/dL

CORRECT COAGULATION

Give:

fresh frozen plasma to replace coagulation factors

platelets* to maintain count >50 × 10⁹/L when bleeding

cryoprecipitate to replace fibrinogen ± factor VIIa

* Platelets may be needed with normal platelet count if aspirin or NSAID taken recently

GIVE OXYGEN
to prevent hypoxaemia

TAKE BLOOD SAMPLES
for coagulation studies + platelets

STOP THE BLEEDING !!
1. Pressure on bleeding site
2. Non-surgical haemostasis (e.g. embolization)
3. Surgical haemostasis

Give clotting factors as required (e.g. VIII in haemophilia)

Give Vitamin K in liver failure + to reverse warfarin (effect<12 h)

Give protamine to reverse heparin effects

Consider aprotinin

RISKS OF TRANSFUSION
1. Acute haemolytic reactions
   - due to incompatible blood group
   - 50% due to administrative error
   - urticaria, rigors, shock, asthma, etc
2. Non-haemolytic reactions (~3%)
   - reaction to donor white cells
   - fever, chills, urticaria
3. Infection
   - viral hepatitis risk ~1% per unit even after testing
4. Acute lung Injury
5. Delayed immune reactions

ADVERSE EFFECTS OF MASSIVE TRANSFUSION
1. Coagulopathy
   e.g. dilutional, DIC
2. Biochemical
   e.g. ↑K⁺, ↓pH, ↓Ca²⁺
3. Hypothermia
4. Volume overload
5. ARDS
6. Infection (hepatitis)

Blood and blood components

Blood is expensive, antigenic and requires cross-matching. Infection risk is reduced by screening blood for HIV, hepatitis, human lymphocytic virus 1, syphilis and CMV. Donated **whole blood** is collected into CPD-A (citrate, phosphate, dextrose-adenine) anticoagulant; one unit is ~430 mL. It is more efficiently stored (i.e. increased shelf-life) and better targeted to individual requirements after division into its various constituents. Centrifugation separates red cells which are resuspended in SAG-M (saline, adenine, glucose: mannitol prevents haemolysis). These **packed red cells** have a haematocrit of ~0.65 and a shelf-life of ~42 days. The platelet-rich plasma fraction (~250 mL) is divided into platelets and plasma. **Platelets** have a shelf-life of ~7 days and one unit increases the platelet count by ~4–9×10^9/L. **Fresh frozen plasma** (FFP) contains all the clotting factors but ~4 units are required for clinically useful increases in serum levels. Storage time is ~12 months. FFP can be further separated into **cryoprecipitate** (factor VIII, fibrinogen) and supernatant (albumin). **Fresh whole blood** is rich in clotting factors and platelets but transfusion reactions are common. It is only used to reduce clotting factor dilution during massive transfusions. **Stored blood** is metabolically active: pH, 2,3-DPG, ATP, platelets and clotting factors decrease, K^+ increases (cell rupture), and microaggregates form.

Coagulation disorders

Coagulation disorders occur when the normal haemostatic balance between **vascular endothelium**, **platelets** and the **clotting–fibrinolytic system** is disrupted. In critical illness the cause is often multifactorial (Fig. c), whereas hereditary disorders stem from a single soluble factor deficiency. **Bleeding disorders** are rapidly identified, as clinical abnormalities are obvious and laboratory monitoring widely available. In contrast, **hypercoagulability** and microvascular thrombosis may not be recognized.

Coagulation tests

Figure (a) illustrates the clotting cascade. **Prothrombin time** (PT) tests the extrinsic pathway including factors II, VII and X which are vitamin K dependent. After addition of tissue thromboplastin and calcium to a sample, clot formation normally occurs within 12–14 s. Causes of prolonged PT are listed in Fig. (a). **Activated partial thromboplastin time** (APPT) tests the intrinsic pathway including factors XII, XI, IX, VIII and X. Following addition of kaolin or phospholipid, coagulation should occur within ~40 s. Figure (a) lists the causes of prolonged APPT. **Platelet counts** <20×10^9/L (<50×10^9/L with coexisting platelet dysfunction) increase the risk of spontaneous bleeding. **Bleeding time** tests platelet function primarily. Following a standard skin incision, bleeding should stop within 9 min. **Activated clotting time**, a bedside test of heparin action, examines clotting in whole blood but is prolonged by thrombocytopenia, hypothermia and fibrinolysis. **Factor assays** (e.g. fibrinogen) are available. **Fibrinogen degradation products** (FDPs) and **D-dimers** are products of fibrinolysis and increase during DIC, sepsis, trauma, VTE and renal failure. FDP assays are widely available. D-dimers are sensitive but not specific for VTE; a negative result reliably excludes VTE (Chapter 27). **PT, APPT and platelet count** detect most acquired bleeding disorders following a detailed history (i.e. previous haemorrhage) and medication review (e.g. aspirin).

Bleeding disorders

- **Genetic coagulopathies.** The haemophilias are sex-linked, recessive diseases causing spontaneous bleeding in affected males. **Haemophilia A** is due to factor VIII deficiency. **Haemophilia B** (Christmas disease) is less common and due to factor IX deficiency. Treatment is with factors VIII and IX, respectively. **Von Willebrand's disease**, an autosomal dominant trait, is the commonest hereditary coagulation disorder. It decreases factor VIII activity and reduces platelet adherence to vascular injury sites. Treatment with DDAVP augments factor VIII and reduces haemorrhagic risk in mild cases. Cryoprecipitate and FFP may be required.
- **Liver disease** causes vitamin K-dependent coagulation factor deficiencies. Rapid correction follows vitamin K therapy except in severe hepatocellular damage. **Vitamin K deficiency** also occurs in malnourished patients and following antibiotic therapy.
- **Anticoagulation agents.** Oral anticoagulants produce vitamin K-dependent clotting factor deficiencies. FFP transiently reverses warfarin-induced anticoagulation whilst vitamin K provides longer-term antagonism. **Heparin** potentiates antithrombin III, which blocks the action of thrombin (±factors IX, X, XI), preventing coagulation and prolonging APPT. It is reversed by protamine sulphate. Cross-reactivity of antibodies against heparin with platelet antigens causes heparin-induced thrombocytopenia (HIT; ~10%) and thrombotic complications. **Antiplatelet agents** (e.g. aspirin) irreversibly inhibit platelet function for ~10 days. **Thrombolysis** may cause haemorrhage (e.g. GI tract). Intracranial bleeding occurs in <0.5–2%. FFP and platelets stop bleeding. **Circulating anticoagulants** develop with some drugs (e.g. penicillin) and diseases (e.g. AIDS, SLE).
- **Disseminated intravascular coagulation** (DIC) follows widespread activation of clotting and fibrinolysis (e.g. sepsis) with concurrent thrombotic and haemorrhagic manifestations. Bleeding is often the presenting symptom. Figure (d) lists the causes of DIC. The underlying cause must be treated, clotting factors and platelets supplemented and low-dose heparin instituted.
- **Thrombocytopenia** is due to decreased production, increased consumption or extracorporeal loss of platelets (Fig. b). Treat the underlying cause (e.g. steroids and immune globulin in ITP, FFP and plasma exchange in TTP).

Transfusion and management of bleeding

A full cross-match procedure takes ~45 min but ABO type determination only ~10 min. O-negative blood (universal donor) is given when blood is needed immediately, but may provoke minor transfusion reactions. Type-specific (ABO-, rhesus-compatible) blood is preferred if time permits. After ~5 units of blood, dilutional clotting disorders and biochemical abnormalities (e.g. hypocalcaemia) develop and may require correction. Blood filters are recommended during large transfusions. Transfusion reactions, effects of massive transfusion (>10 units/24 h) and management of bleeding are illustrated in Fig. (e).

Hypercoagulable disorders

Thromboembolism (Chapter 27) involves a predisposing genetic disorder in ~20% of cases (e.g. antithrombin III, protein C and S deficiency and lupus anticoagulant). A family history of thrombosis, recurrent clotting episodes, unusual sites (e.g. arms) and recurrent spontaneous abortions are suggestive.

42 Drug overdose and poisoning

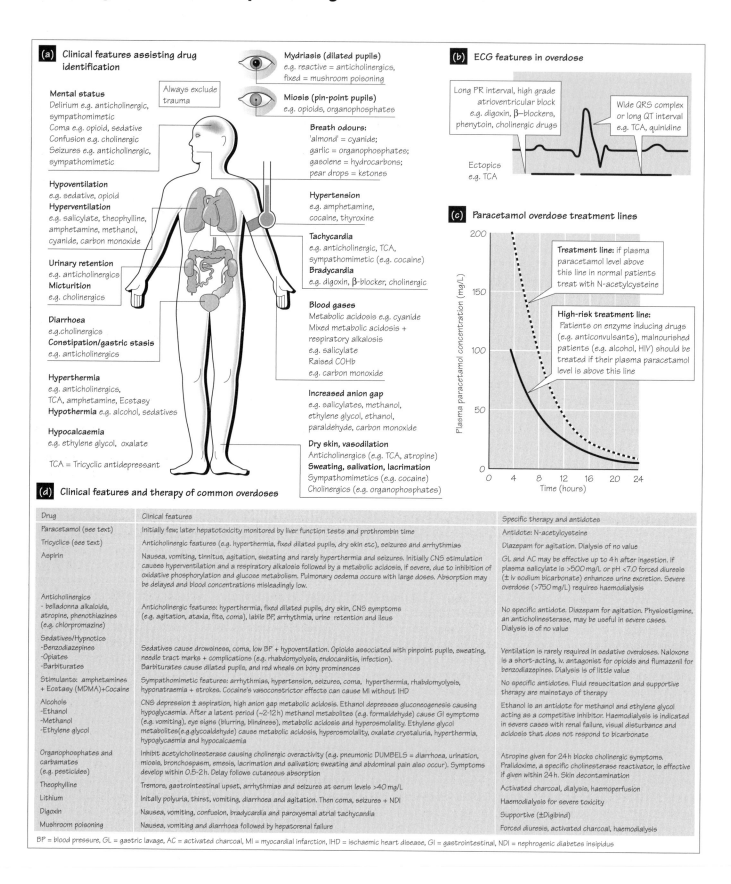

(a) Clinical features assisting drug identification

Always exclude trauma

Mental status
Delirium e.g. anticholinergic, sympathomimetic
Coma e.g. opioid, sedative
Confusion e.g. cholinergic
Seizures e.g. anticholinergic, sympathomimetic

Hypoventilation
e.g. sedative, opioid
Hyperventilation
e.g. salicylate, theophylline, amphetamine, methanol, cyanide, carbon monoxide

Urinary retention
e.g. anticholinergics
Micturition
e.g. cholinergics

Diarrhoea
e.g. cholinergics
Constipation/gastric stasis
e.g. anticholinergics

Hyperthermia
e.g. anticholinergics, TCA, amphetamine, Ecstasy
Hypothermia e.g. alcohol, sedatives

Hypocalcaemia
e.g. ethylene glycol, oxalate

TCA = Tricyclic antidepressant

Mydriasis (dilated pupils)
e.g. reactive = anticholinergics, fixed = mushroom poisoning

Miosis (pin-point pupils)
e.g. opioids, organophosphates

Breath odours:
'almond' = cyanide;
garlic = organophosphates;
gasolene = hydrocarbons;
pear drops = ketones

Hypertension
e.g. amphetamine, cocaine, thyroxine

Tachycardia
e.g. anticholinergic, TCA, sympathomimetic (e.g. cocaine)
Bradycardia
e.g. digoxin, β-blocker, cholinergic

Blood gases
Metabolic acidosis e.g. cyanide
Mixed metabolic acidosis + respiratory alkalosis e.g. salicylate
Raised COHb e.g. carbon monoxide

Increased anion gap
e.g. salicylates, methanol, ethylene glycol, ethanol, paraldehyde, carbon monoxide

Dry skin, vasodilation
Anticholinergics (e.g. TCA, atropine)
Sweating, salivation, lacrimation
Sympathomimetics (e.g. cocaine)
Cholinergics (e.g. organophosphates)

(b) ECG features in overdose

Long PR interval, high grade atrioventricular block e.g. digoxin, β-blockers, phenytoin, cholinergic drugs

Wide QRS complex or long QT interval e.g. TCA, quinidine

Ectopics e.g. TCA

(c) Paracetamol overdose treatment lines

Treatment line: if plasma paracetamol level above this line in normal patients treat with N-acetylcysteine

High-risk treatment line: Patients on enzyme inducing drugs (e.g. anticonvulsants), malnourished patients (e.g. alcohol, HIV) should be treated if their plasma paracetamol level is above this line

(d) Clinical features and therapy of common overdoses

Drug	Clinical features	Specific therapy and antidotes
Paracetamol (see text)	Initially few; later hepatotoxicity monitored by liver function tests and prothrombin time	Antidote: N-acetylcysteine
Tricyclics (see text)	Anticholinergic features (e.g. hyperthermia, fixed dilated pupils, dry skin etc.), seizures and arrhythmias	Diazepam for agitation. Dialysis of no value
Aspirin	Nausea, vomiting, tinnitus, agitation, sweating and rarely hyperthermia and seizures. Initially CNS stimulation causes hyperventilation and a respiratory alkalosis followed by a metabolic acidosis, if severe, due to inhibition of oxidative phosphorylation and glucose metabolism. Pulmonary oedema occurs with large doses. Absorption may be delayed and blood concentrations misleadingly low.	GL and AC may be effective up to 4h after ingestion. If plasma salicylate is >500mg/L or pH <7.0 forced diuresis (± iv sodium bicarbonate) enhances urine excretion. Severe overdose (>750mg/L) requires haemodialysis
Anticholinergics - belladonna alkaloids, atropine, phenothiazines (e.g. chlorpromazine)	Anticholinergic features: hyperthermia, fixed dilated pupils, dry skin, CNS symptoms (e.g. agitation, ataxia, fits, coma), labile BP, arrhythmia, urine retention and ileus	No specific antidote. Diazepam for agitation. Physiostigmine, an anticholinesterase, may be useful in severe cases. Dialysis is of no value
Sedatives/Hypnotics -Benzodiazepines -Opiates -Barbiturates	Sedatives cause drowsiness, coma, low BP + hypoventilation. Opioids associated with pinpoint pupils, sweating, needle tract marks + complications (e.g. rhabdomyolysis, endocarditis, infection). Barbiturates cause dilated pupils, and red wheals on bony prominences	Ventilation is rarely required in sedative overdoses. Naloxone is a short-acting, iv. antagonist for opioids and flumazenil for benzodiazepines. Dialysis is of little value
Stimulants: amphetamines + Ecstasy (MDMA)+Cocaine	Sympathomimetic features: arrhythmias, hypertension, seizures, coma, hyperthermia, rhabdomyolysis, hyponatraemia + strokes. Cocaine's vasoconstrictor effects can cause MI without IHD	No specific antidotes. Fluid resuscitation and supportive therapy are mainstays of therapy
Alcohols -Ethanol -Methanol -Ethylene glycol	CNS depression ± aspiration, high anion gap metabolic acidosis. Ethanol depresses gluconeogenesis causing hypoglycaemia. After a latent period (~2-12h) methanol metabolites (e.g. formaldehyde) cause GI symptoms (e.g. vomiting), eye signs (blurring, blindness), metabolic acidosis and hyperosmolality. Ethylene glycol metabolites (e.g.glycoaldehyde) cause metabolic acidosis, hyperosmolality, oxalate crystaluria, hyperthermia, hypoglycaemia and hypocalcaemia	Ethanol is an antidote for methanol and ethylene glycol acting as a competitive inhibitor. Haemodialysis is indicated in severe cases with renal failure, visual disturbance and acidosis that does not respond to bicarbonate
Organophosphates and carbamates (e.g. pesticides)	Inhibit acetylcholinesterase causing cholinergic overactivity (e.g. pneumonic DUMBELS = diarrhoea, urination, miosis, bronchospasm, emesis, lacrimation and salivation; sweating and abdominal pain also occur). Symptoms develop within 0.5-2h. Delay follows cutaneous absorption	Atropine given for 24h blocks cholinergic symptoms. Pralidoxime, a specific cholinesterase reactivator, is effective if given within 24h. Skin decontamination
Theophylline	Tremors, gastrointestinal upset, arrhythmias and seizures at serum levels >40mg/L	Activated charcoal, dialysis, haemoperfusion
Lithium	Initally polyuria, thirst, vomiting, diarrhoea and agitation. Then coma, seizures + NDI	Haemodialysis for severe toxicity
Digoxin	Nausea, vomiting, confusion, bradycardia and paroxysmal atrial tachycardia	Supportive (±Digibind)
Mushroom poisoning	Nausea, vomiting and diarrhoea followed by hepatorenal failure	Forced diuresis, activated charcoal, haemodialysis

BP = blood pressure, GL = gastric lavage, AC = activated charcoal, MI = myocardial infarction, IHD = ischaemic heart disease, GI = gastrointestinal, NDI = nephrogenic diabetes insipidus

Overdoses and poisonings account for ~10% of hospital and ~15% of critical care unit admissions. Self-administration of a few drugs (e.g. paracetamol, tricyclic antidepressants) accounts for ~90–95% of adult acute poisonings. In-hospital mortality is <1% as most deaths occur before admission due to arrhythmia or respiratory arrest. Most episodes are 'a cry for help' rather than genuine suicide attempts and occur in young people (<35 years old; M : F 1 : 1.5) with a history of similar episodes. Fatal overdoses are more likely in patients >45 years old with serious suicidal intent. In children, poisoning is usually accidental due to ingestion of a single agent.

In general, routine support and prevention of absorption are more important than active measures to hasten drug elimination. A practical approach to overdose management requires:

1 *Resuscitation and supportive care* including airways protection, respiratory support, fluid resuscitation and acid–base balance. Prolonged unconsciousness is often associated with hypothermia, aspiration of gastric contents, pressure necrosis of muscle and compartment syndrome. Drug-induced hyperthermia (e.g. salicylates, anticholinergics) is uncommon (Chapter 15).

2 *Substance identification.* Although **history** is unreliable, important information includes *drugs taken* (±time taken, dosage, route), *past history* (i.e. previous attempts), *circumstances* (e.g. witnesses, empty containers, syringes) and *associated trauma.*

- **Examination** (Fig. a) provides important diagnostic clues.
- **Investigations** (Figs a and b) include drug identification (e.g. blood, urine, gastric aspirates), routine paracetamol, aspirin and alcohol levels in unconscious patients, blood counts, coagulation profiles, biochemistry including liver function tests, serum osmolality (e.g. methanol, ethylene glycol), blood gases and anion gap (Chapter 12), CXR (e.g. pulmonary oedema with salicylates) and ECG (e.g. myocardial ischaemia with cocaine).

3 *Prevention of absorption* is controversial, but best achieved by gastric lavage followed by instillation of activated charcoal.

- **Gastric lavage (GL)** should be performed in most serious overdoses, up to 4 h after ingestion. Useful recovery of drugs which impair gastric emptying (e.g. anticholinergics), form concretions (e.g. theophylline) or are delayed release preparations (e.g. salicylates) may be achieved later. GL is not effective for alcohol and is harmful after caustic or petroleum product ingestion. Lavage is performed in the left lateral decubitus position using a large orogastric (Ewald) tube that facilitates removal of pill fragments. The airway must be protected as aspiration of gastric contents is the main complication. Oropharyngeal trauma and oesophageal perforation can occur.
- **Activated charcoal (AC)** is an effective adsorbent and promotes drug elimination (e.g. salicylates, theophylline). It is given after GL and at 4-h intervals. AC does not bind iron, lithium, alcohols, acids, alkalis, cyanide or organophosphates (e.g. pesticides). It causes constipation and may be given with added cathartic (e.g. sorbitol) as an aqueous slurry.
- **Additional measures** include: (i) **induced vomiting** (e.g. ipecac) which is rarely indicated and risks aspiration or oesophageal tears. It is contraindicated in obtunded patients, children <6 months old and following caustic agents or hydrocarbons; (ii) **cathartics** promote diarrhoea and reduced drug absorption but risk fluid and electrolyte loss; (iii) **skin**

decontamination is essential for transdermally absorbed toxins (e.g. organophosphates); and (iv) **endoscopy/surgery** are rarely necessary (e.g. iron overdose, body packers).

4 *Enhanced drug elimination* is only indicated in life-threatening poisoning as some techniques have associated risks.

- **Gut dialysis** uses repeated doses of AC to bind drugs with an enterohepatic circulation which are excreted in bile (e.g. theophylline, digoxin, carbamazepine).
- **Forced diuresis** enhances drug excretion by increasing urine production to 2–5 mL/kg/h with intravenous fluid (±diuretic) but risks fluid overload. Alkalinization with sodium bicarbonate promotes salicylate, tricyclic antidepressant and barbiturate excretion but is only used in severe cases.
- **Haemodialysis** removes low molecular weight, water-soluble molecules, with a small volume of distribution and low protein binding (e.g. salicylates, methanol, theophylline).
- **Haemoperfusion** using charcoal or resin columns is useful for lipid-soluble drugs (e.g. theophylline, barbiturates) but may cause hypocalcaemia and coagulopathy.

Specific management

Figure (d) summarizes the clinical features and management of overdoses and poisonings. Paracetamol and tricyclic antidepressants are most common, often in combination with alcohol.

- **Paracetamol** overdose (POD) depletes hepatic glutathione stores, causing accumulation of a hydroxylamine metabolite which causes liver and renal damage. Patients taking anticonvulsants or with alcohol dependency are at greater risk of hepatotoxicity. Treatment with N-acetylcysteine (NAC) raises glutathione levels and reduces toxicity. POD causes 200 deaths/year in the UK and ≥15 g can be lethal. Initially there are few symptoms apart from nausea, vomiting and abdominal pain. Signs and biochemical evidence of hepatocellular necrosis present after 24 h and peak at 3–4 days. The recovery phase lasts ~8 days. Initial management includes GL and AC up to 4 h after a significant POD. Intravenous NAC is administered if paracetamol levels measured at 4 h are above the treatment line (Fig. c) or if >10 g has been ingested. NAC is most effective when given within 12 h. Rapid administration can cause bronchospasm, urticaria and anaphylaxis. Methionine is an oral alternative to NAC. Early referral to a liver unit is appropriate if liver failure develops. Liver transplantation may be indicated in established liver failure.
- **Tricyclic antidepressants** (TCAs) cause most overdose fatalities (~300 deaths/year in the UK) but in-hospital mortality is still <1%. Toxicity is due to anticholinergic effects which cause fixed dilated pupils, dry red skin, hyperthermia, tachycardia, urine retention and CNS hyperreactivity (e.g. psychosis, hallucinations, seizures). Severely intoxicated patients are accurately described as 'hot as a hare, blind as a bat, dry as a bone and mad as a hatter'. There is no specific antidote. GL and AC are essential due to associated ileus, delayed gastric emptying and enterohepatic circulation. The ECG signals cardiac and CNS toxicity when the QRS complex is >0.12 s. Potentially life-threatening arrhythmias and hypotension respond to correction of hypoxia, acidosis and cardioversion but can be very resistant to antiarrhythmic agents. Lidocaine and phenytoin are the most beneficial antiarrhythmics. Type 1a drugs (e.g. quinidine) further impair conduction and should be avoided. Recovery occurs in ~24 h due to rapid metabolism.

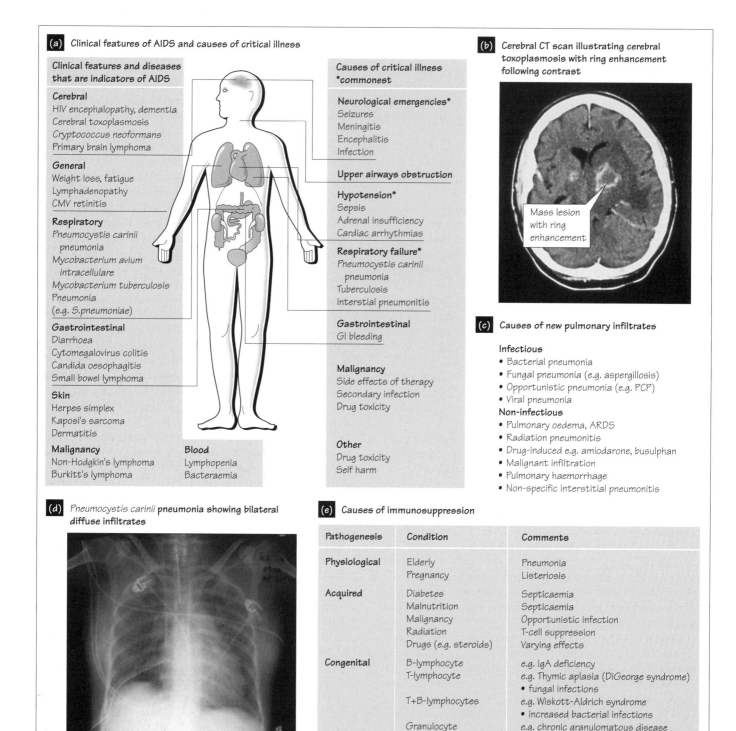

(a) Clinical features of AIDS and causes of critical illness

Clinical features and diseases that are indicators of AIDS

Cerebral
HIV encephalopathy, dementia
Cerebral toxoplasmosis
Cryptococcus neoformans
Primary brain lymphoma

General
Weight loss, fatigue
Lymphadenopathy
CMV retinitis

Respiratory
Pneumocystis carinii
 pneumonia
Mycobacterium avium
 intracellulare
Mycobacterium tuberculosis
Pneumonia
(e.g. S.pneumoniae)

Gastrointestinal
Diarrhoea
Cytomegalovirus colitis
Candida oesophagitis
Small bowel lymphoma

Skin
Herpes simplex
Kaposi's sarcoma
Dermatitis

Malignancy
Non-Hodgkin's lymphoma
Burkitt's lymphoma

Blood
Lymphopenia
Bacteraemia

Causes of critical illness
***commonest**

Neurological emergencies*
Seizures
Meningitis
Encephalitis
Infection

Upper airways obstruction

Hypotension*
Sepsis
Adrenal insufficiency
Cardiac arrhythmias

Respiratory failure*
Pneumocystis carinii
 pneumonia
Tuberculosis
Interstial pneumonitis

Gastrointestinal
GI bleeding

Malignancy
Side effects of therapy
Secondary infection
Drug toxicity

Other
Drug toxicity
Self harm

(b) Cerebral CT scan illustrating cerebral toxoplasmosis with ring enhancement following contrast

Mass lesion with ring enhancement

(c) Causes of new pulmonary infiltrates

Infectious
• Bacterial pneumonia
• Fungal pneumonia (e.g. aspergillosis)
• Opportunistic pneumonia (e.g. PCP)
• Viral pneumonia
Non-infectious
• Pulmonary oedema, ARDS
• Radiation pneumonitis
• Drug-induced e.g. amiodarone, busulphan
• Malignant infiltration
• Pulmonary haemorrhage
• Non-specific interstitial pneumonitis

(d) Pneumocystis carinii pneumonia showing bilateral diffuse infiltrates

(e) Causes of immunosuppression

Pathogenesis	Condition	Comments
Physiological	Elderly	Pneumonia
	Pregnancy	Listeriosis
Acquired	Diabetes	Septicaemia
	Malnutrition	Septicaemia
	Malignancy	Opportunistic infection
	Radiation	T-cell suppression
	Drugs (e.g. steroids)	Varying effects
Congenital	B-lymphocyte	e.g. IgA deficiency
	T-lymphocyte	e.g. Thymic aplasia (DiGeorge syndrome)
		• fungal infections
	T+B-lymphocytes	e.g. Wiskott-Aldrich syndrome
		• increased bacterial infections
	Granulocyte	e.g. chronic granulomatous disease
		• staphylococcal infection
	Complement	e.g. C2, C3
		• septicaemia
Others	Cystic fibrosis	Viscid sputum
		• pneumonia

General factors

Malnutrition, disease (e.g. diabetes, malignancy) and medical interventions impair the immune system and risk critical illness due to **infectious** and **non-infectious** (e.g. neoplasia, drug reactions, haemorrhage, graft vs. host disease, respiratory failure) causes (Fig. e). Primary failure of **T-lymphocyte** (cell-mediated) function predisposes to viral or fungal infections and neoplasia. **B-lymphocyte** (antibody-mediated; 'humoral') disorders and **granulocytopenia** are associated with bacterial infections. Fever in profoundly neutropenic (<1000 granulocytes/mm³) patients is an emergency, particularly when due to infection, and survival depends on rapid diagnosis and treatment. Unfortunately, infection with commensal organisms (e.g. *Pneumocystis*, *Aspergillus*) and lack of localized inflammation often make diagnosis difficult. Primary bacteraemia and soft tissue (e.g. perirectal abscess) infections are characteristic, although any site may be infected. **Pulmonary infiltrates** do not always indicate infection, as there are many non-infective causes (Fig. c). Establishing the diagnosis may require invasive techniques (e.g. open lung biopsy) with associated risks (e.g. poor healing, haemorrhage).

General management

Survival of febrile neutropenic patients depends on **early empirical antibiotic therapy** effective against potential infecting organisms including Gram-negative rods (e.g. *Pseudomonas*), staphylococci and fungi (e.g. *Aspergillus*). Impaired cell-mediated immunity predisposes to *Pneumocystis* and *Candida* infection. **Cultures** of blood, urine, sputum and skin lesions must be obtained before starting **broad-spectrum antibiotics** including extended-spectrum penicillins, third-generation cephalosporins and aminoglycosides and in some cases cover against methicillin-resistant *Staphylococcus aureus* (MRSA) infections. Many centres advocate the addition of **antifungal therapy** (e.g. amphotericin) if fever persists for >72 h after starting antibiotics.

Specific causes

Acquired immunodeficiency syndrome (AIDS) is caused by human immunodeficiency virus (HIV) which infects, replicates within, impairs and eventually depletes CD₄ T lymphocytes. HIV is transmitted by sexual contact, in blood products, during pregnancy from mother to child and through breast milk. Over 30 million people are infected worldwide. AIDS is defined as HIV-infected individuals with a CD₄ count <200/mL of blood (or a CD₄ count <14% of all lymphocytes). Low CD₄ counts are associated with clinical features, diseases and critical illnesses which are indicators of AIDS (Fig. a).
- *Pneumocystis carinii* **pneumonia (PCP)** with respiratory failure is most common but the incidence has decreased with prophylactic Septrin therapy.

  Clinical features include fever, dry cough and dyspnoea. Pneumothorax occurs in ~2% of cases.

  Investigations demonstrate impaired diffusion capacity on lung function testing, desaturation during exercise and generalized alveolitis. Chest radiography typically shows bilateral interstitial infiltrates (Fig. d) but may be normal or focally consolidated. Giemsa, silver and immunofluorescent stains of sputum, particularly when induced using nebulized 3 N saline, detects pneumocysts in >70% of cases. Bronchoscopic washings detect >90% of cases, with transbronchial lung biopsies the most reliable technique.

  Treatment is with high-dose intravenous co-trimoxazole (Septrin), which can cause severe skin rashes (~30%), vomiting, colitis and hepatitis. Alternative therapy with pentamidine also causes side-effects. High-dose steroids reduce alveolitis, respiratory failure and mortality.
- **Other opportunistic infections** include pulmonary tuberculosis, toxoplasmosis (Fig. b), candidiasis, *Cryptococcus neoformans*, CMV and herpes simplex. HIV-infected patients with undiagnosed respiratory illness should be isolated until TB has been excluded.

Hospital precautions. Assume all patients are HIV positive and take appropriate measures (e.g. gloves, masks). The infection risk following HIV-contaminated needlestick injury is ~0.3%. After cleansing, seek expert advice and start prophylactic therapy.

Malignant disease, particularly haematological and lymphoproliferative disorders, is increasingly associated with improved long-term prognosis. Potentially reversible life-threatening complications due to the tumour (e.g. hypercalcaemia) or treatment (e.g. chemotherapy) may require admission to critical care facilities. Such patients are susceptible to infection due to the profound leucopenia that occurs 10–14 days after aggressive chemotherapy or bone marrow transplantation, disease-mediated immunosuppression (e.g. impaired lymphocyte function) and invasive procedures (e.g. line insertion). In general, mortality rates are high (>70%) when patients with malignant disease develop acute illnesses, but prolonged, high quality survival justifies aggressive management in selected cases.

Postsplenectomy infection may be fatal as loss of splenic phagocytic function allows rapid bacterial proliferation. Infection is usually due to encapsulated bacteria (e.g. pneumococci, *Haemophilus*). Prophylactic antibiotics (e.g. penicillin) and vaccination against influenza, pneumococcus, *H. influenzae* and meningococcus are recommended.

Systemic disease may increase the risk of infection (e.g. diabetes, malnutrition). **Cirrhosis** impairs hepatic phagocytic function. **Connective tissue diseases** (e.g. SLE) are associated with immunosuppression due to the effects of therapy (e.g. steroids, cyclophosphamide) and low white cell counts. **Primary immunodeficiency disorders** (e.g. DiGeorge syndrome) rarely cause sepsis or critical illness.

Transplant surgery requires postoperative immunosuppressive therapy (e.g. cyclosporin, steroids, azathioprine) to prevent graft vs. host organ rejection. Cyclosporin is more specifically directed against T cells than B cells, is less immunosuppressive and has greater antirejection potency than azathioprine. Since its introduction infections have decreased and graft survival has increased. The greatest risk of rejection is in the first 6–12 weeks following transplant after which the body develops a degree of tolerance to the graft and the cyclosporin dosage can be reduced. During this period of maximal T-cell suppression, renal transplant recipients are prone to CMV, cryptococcus, PCP, herpes simplex and *Aspergillus* infections. Longer term there is a continuing risk from opportunistic infections and a slightly increased risk of malignancy (e.g. non-Hodgkin's lymphoma).

Immunosuppressive therapy is required for many common disorders (e.g. Crohn's disease, rheumatoid arthritis). These medications (e.g. steroids, cyclophosphamide, azathioprine, methotrexate) and other therapies (e.g. radiotherapy) cause immunosuppression and are associated with increased infection risk.

44 Trauma

(a) Manual in-line cervical immobilization

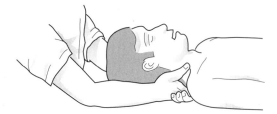

(b) Cervical radiograph of a potentially unstable fracture in a 22-year-old following a road traffic accident

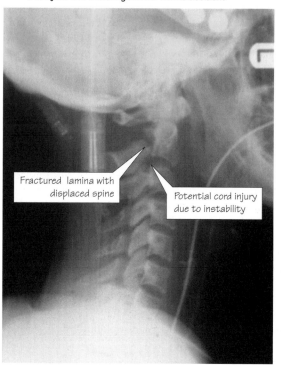

Fractured lamina with displaced spine

Potential cord injury due to instability

(c) Classification of haemorrhage severity

Class	Circulating volume loss	Approx volume loss (70 kg man)	Clinical signs
Class 1	<15%	<750 mL	Minimal signs
Class 2	15-30%	<1500 mL	↑HR + ↓BP; sweating ↓pulse pressure
Class 3	30-40%	<2000 mL	Agitated, sweating, oliguria, ↑HR (>120/min) ↓BP (systolic ~90 mmHg)
Class 4	>40%	>2000 mL	Preterminal, drowsy ↓BP (systolic <90 mmHg)

(d) Types of cervical fracture (#)

Fractured odontoid process:

AP view through mouth　　Lateral view in extension

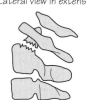

Cord damage is often mild but traction is usually required and surgery if the fracture does not unite

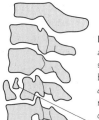

Burst fractures:
are very painful. They are stable unless there is bony displacement. Cord damage is unusual. They require support in a collar until fusion occurs

Hyperextension injury:
radiographs appear normal because the posterior ligament is intact. These # are stable in the neutral position and can be treated with a collar. Instability may occur in hyperextension

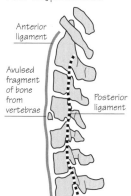

Anterior ligament

Avulsed fragment of bone from vertebrae

Posterior ligament

Anterior dislocations:
disrupt the posterior ligament and are therefore unstable. Injury is often minimal but tetraplegia can occur. Treatment is immediate reduction using skull traction with fusion 3-4 weeks later

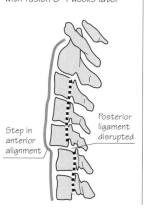

Step in anterior alignment

Posterior ligament disrupted

Fracture dislocations:
cause the most serious neck injuries and usually occur at C$_{5/6}$ and C$_{6/7}$. They are very unstable and can damage the spinal cord. The safest treatment is continuous skull traction for 4-6 weeks followed by fusion

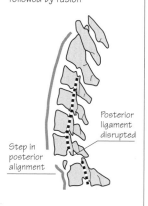

Posterior ligament disrupted

Step in posterior alignment

Trauma is the leading cause of death in young people (<40 years old). **The Advanced Trauma Life Support (ATLS) Programme** recommends a **structured approach** to management, by a well organized **trauma team**, in which the greatest risk to life is treated first and lack of a definitive diagnosis does not delay appropriate therapy. The airways, breathing, circulation (ABC) system recognizes that **airways obstruction** is more rapidly fatal than **inadequate ventilation**, which is more serious than **loss of circulating volume**. The next most dangerous problem is an expanding **intracranial mass lesion**. Although early resuscitation reduces morbidity and mortality, **prehospital treatment** is limited to ensuring adequate oxygenation, ventilation and spinal immobilization. Fluid resuscitation should not delay transfer to hospital. The sequence of trauma management is as follows.

Primary survey and resuscitation

- **Airway and cervical spine control.** All trauma victims require supplemental oxygen and spinal immobilization with manual in-line cervical stabilization (MILS; Fig. a) or a hard cervical collar, sandbags and tape. Establish a patent upper airway (e.g. remove foreign bodies, oropharyngeal airway) and assess laryngeal reflexes (Chapter 7). If the airway is at risk, intubation by rapid sequence induction with MILS and cricoid pressure is necessary (Chapter 9). Profound hypotension may occur with anaesthetic induction in hypovolaemic patients.
- **Breathing.** Treat immediate life-threatening chest injuries (e.g. pneumothorax, massive haemothorax, flail chest) and anticipate the increased risk of pneumothorax (±tension) associated with mechanical ventilation (MV) in these patients (Chapters 10, 46). Prophylactic MV is required in head-injured patients at risk from hypoxia, hypercapnia and BP fluctuations (Chapter 45).
- **Circulation.** Initially control major external haemorrhage by direct pressure, establish intravenous access with large-bore peripheral or central (e.g. femoral) cannulae and institute ECG monitoring. Early hypotension is usually due to hypovolaemia but other causes include myocardial contusion, aortic rupture, tension pneumothorax, neurogenic shock and cardiac tamponade (secondary survey). Clinical signs and volume of blood loss are used to classify hypovolaemia (Fig. c). In healthy young patients hypotension and shock are not observed until >30% loss of circulating volume. Early fluid replacement, guided by appropriate monitoring, prevents tissue ischaemia and subsequent organ dysfunction (Chapters 2, 4, 5, 41). Fluid is warmed as hypothermia will increase bleeding and mortality. Blood should be administered when haemocrit is <0.3 or haemoglobin <10g/dL. **Immediate surgery** may be required to control bleeding.
- **Neurological status.** Record pupillary light responses and GCS (Chapters 37, 45).
- **General management.** Fully undress the patient to facilitate examination but avoid aggravating hypothermia. Catheterization to monitor urine output follows exclusion of urethral injury. In basal skull fractures, nasogastric tubes may cause meningeal infection. The orogastric route is preferred.

Secondary survey and definitive treatment

Detailed clinical examination and referral for specialist therapy follow resuscitation.
- **Head and face** are inspected for lacerations, haematomas, depressed fractures, eye and orbit injury and mobile midface or mandible segments. Clinical features of basal skull fracture include racoon eyes, bruising over the mastoids (Battle's sign), subhyaloid haemorrhage, haemotympanium and CSF rhinorrhoea or otorrhoea. Head injury is discussed in Chapter 45.
- **Chest** examination may detect potentially life-threatening tracheobronchial injuries, pulmonary or cardiac contusion, aortic rupture, oesophageal and diaphragmatic rupture. Management is discussed in Chapter 46.
- **Abdomen.** Concealed intra-abdominal bleeding or viscus perforation should be considered if shock persists despite fluid re-placement. Accompanying abdominal bruising, lacerations, tenderness and distension are frequently detected. Rectal examination may reveal reduced perianal sensation and anal sphincter tone in spinal injury, bleeding after bowel injury and a high prostate with urethral injury. Abdominal ultrasound, CT scan, diagnostic peritoneal lavage and occasionally laparotomy are indicated when examination is unreliable in unconscious, ventilated or persistently hypotensive patients. Cardiovascular instability often precludes transfer for CT scans.
- **Spinal injury** occurs in ~2% of major trauma victims (Fig. b). Most injuries occur in the cervical region (~50%). The commonest sites are C_5/C_6, C_6/C_7 and T_{12}/L_1.

Examination. Motor or sensory function below the cord lesion on neurological assessment has prognostic implications and must be recorded. The patient is carefully log-rolled to allow palpation of the spine for tenderness and 'step-off' deformity (Fig. d).

Investigations. Cervical (e.g. lateral, anteroposterior (AP) and open-mouth views), thoracic and lumbar spine X-rays are essential although injury may occur *without radiographic abnormality*. CT scans assess injured regions and areas not clearly visualized on X-ray. MRI scans demonstrate ligament and cord damage.

Management prevents secondary cord damage by immobilization and adequate resuscitation prevents spinal cord ischaemia.

Early steroids may improve long-term outcome.

Spinal stability. Disruption of the posterior ligamentous complex produces an unstable spine. Early referral for fixation is advocated by many specialist centres. Potentially unstable cervical fractures (Fig. d) may require temporary stabilization with a halo frame.

Respiration. Cord lesions above C_4 inhibit diaphragmatic function and always require ventilatory support. Intercostal muscles are innervated by T_2–T_{12} and patients with lesions above this level are dependent on diaphragmatic breathing with decreased tidal volumes and impaired cough.

Circulation. Initial cord injury causes massive sympathetic outflow with severe hypertension. Subsequent loss of sympathetic tone causes neurogenic shock (Chapter 4). Lesions above T_1 prevent sympathetic reflex tachycardia, which limits the cardiovascular stress response, and profound bradycardia may follow vagal stimulation (e.g. bronchial suctioning).

Neurology. Spinal shock describes muscle flaccidity and areflexia following spinal injury. It lasts for 2–70 days and muscle contractures and spasms may follow resolution. Autonomic dysreflexia occurs with cord injuries above T_7 (~65%). Stimulation below the level of the lesion (e.g. bladder distension) causes a sympathetic reflex with flushing, hypertension and bradycardia that may precipitate seizures or strokes. **General factors** include hypothermia due to vasodilation, paralytic ileus and bladder atony requiring catheterization. Meticulous nursing avoids pressure sores.

Peripheral trauma

Long-bone fractures are associated with occult haemorrhage and neurovascular injuries which must be detected and treated. Crush injuries may result in compartment syndrome requiring decompressive fasciotomy. Associated rhabdomyolysis causes hypovolaemia, hyperkalaemia and renal failure unless preventative measures are instituted (Chapter 31).

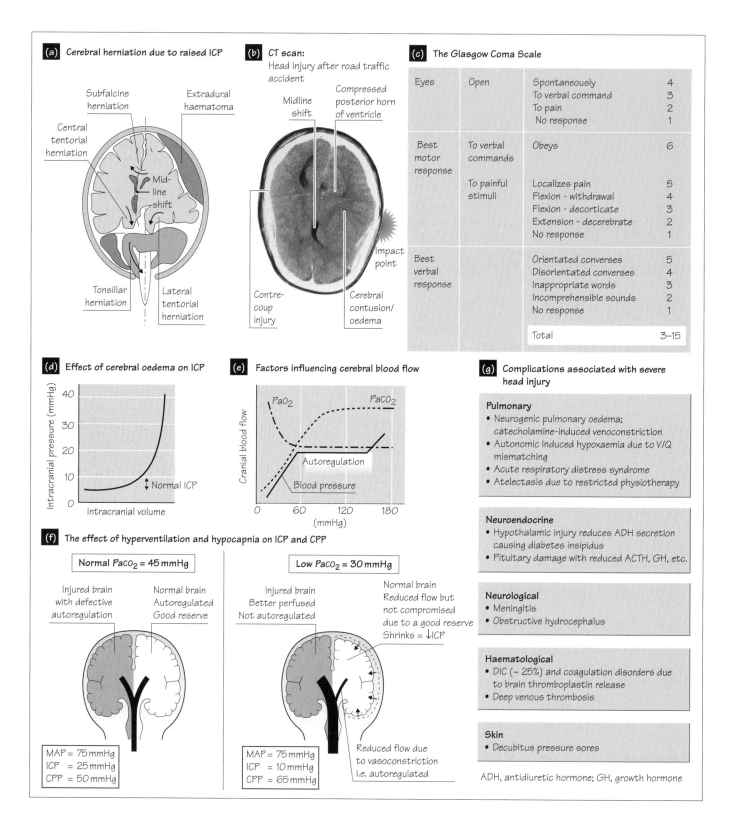

(a) Cerebral herniation due to raised ICP

Subfalcine herniation · Extradural haematoma · Central tentorial herniation · Mid-line shift · Tonsillar herniation · Lateral tentorial herniation

(b) CT scan:
Head injury after road traffic accident

Midline shift · Compressed posterior horn of ventricle · Contre-coup injury · Cerebral contusion/oedema · Impact point

(c) The Glasgow Coma Scale

Eyes	Open	Spontaneously	4
		To verbal command	3
		To pain	2
		No response	1
Best motor response	To verbal commands	Obeys	6
	To painful stimuli	Localizes pain	5
		Flexion - withdrawal	4
		Flexion - decorticate	3
		Extension - decerebrate	2
		No response	1
Best verbal response		Orientated converses	5
		Disorientated converses	4
		Inappropriate words	3
		Incomprehensible sounds	2
		No response	1
Total			3–15

(d) Effect of cerebral oedema on ICP

Intracranial pressure (mmHg) vs Intracranial volume. Normal ICP marked.

(e) Factors influencing cerebral blood flow

PaO_2 · $PaCO_2$ · Cranial blood flow · Autoregulation · Blood pressure · 0, 60, 120, 180 (mmHg)

(f) The effect of hyperventilation and hypocapnia on ICP and CPP

Normal $PaCO_2$ = 45 mmHg

Injured brain with defective autoregulation · Normal brain Autoregulated Good reserve

MAP = 75 mmHg
ICP = 25 mmHg
CPP = 50 mmHg

Low $PaCO_2$ = 30 mmHg

Injured brain Better perfused Not autoregulated · Normal brain Reduced flow but not compromised due to a good reserve Shrinks = ↓ICP

Reduced flow due to vasoconstriction i.e. autoregulated

MAP = 75 mmHg
ICP = 10 mmHg
CPP = 65 mmHg

(g) Complications associated with severe head injury

Pulmonary
- Neurogenic pulmonary oedema; catecholamine-induced venoconstriction
- Autonomic induced hypoxaemia due to V/Q mismatching
- Acute respiratory distress syndrome
- Atelectasis due to restricted physiotherapy

Neuroendocrine
- Hypothalamic injury reduces ADH secretion causing diabetes insipidus
- Pituitary damage with reduced ACTH, GH, etc.

Neurological
- Meningitis
- Obstructive hydrocephalus

Haematological
- DIC (~ 25%) and coagulation disorders due to brain thromboplastin release
- Deep venous thrombosis

Skin
- Decubitus pressure sores

ADH, antidiuretic hormone; GH, growth hormone

Head injury accounts for ~33% of trauma deaths. Road traffic accidents, falls, assaults and gunshot wounds account for most serious head injuries. Two mechanisms cause neural tissue damage.

1 *Primary injury* is sustained during trauma and includes brain lacerations, contusions and diffuse axonal injury due to shear forces during acceleration or deceleration. It is irreversible.

2 *Secondary injury* (Figs a and b) is due to **raised intracranial pressure** (ICP) and **inadequate cerebral perfusion**. It accounts for ~50% of deaths and therapeutic intervention improves outcome. Causes are: **(i) intracranial,** including cerebral oedema, hydrocephalus, space-occupying lesions (SOLs, e.g. extradural haemorrhage), cerebral ischaemia (e.g. vasospasm, seizures, vascular distortion) and inflammatory mediators; and **(ii) systemic,** including hypotension, hypoxia, anaemia, hyper-/hypoglycaemia, hyperthermia and hyper-/hypocapnia.

Pathophysiology

The skull is a fixed volume containing brain, blood and CSF. Initially cerebral oedema (±SOL) displaces blood and CSF with little effect on normal ICP (~5–10mmHg). Further swelling rapidly raises ICP (Fig. d). After trauma, ICP peaks at ~72h and may cause cerebral herniation (Fig. a). Increased ICP (e.g. >25mmHg) reflects the severity of brain injury but reduced **cerebral perfusion pressure (CPP)**, which is the difference between mean arterial pressure (MAP) and ICP, is more important, as this impairs cerebral blood flow (CBF) causing ischaemia. Therapy should aim to maintain a normal CPP (i.e. >60mmHg) as neural dysfunction occurs at <40mmHg and neuronal death at <20mmHg.

Normally CBF is independent of blood pressure (i.e. autoregulated) but is sensitive to P_aO_2 and P_aCO_2 (Fig. e). In injured brain autoregulation fails and perfusion directly parallels CPP.
Hypoxia or hypercapnia dilates normal vessels and diverts blood flow away from damaged cerebral tissue. The associated increase in cerebral blood volume (CBV) raises ICP, reduces CPP and CBF, and further aggravates ischaemia in damaged brain tissue.
Hypocapnia (Fig. f) constricts normal vessels, reducing CBV and ICP. This increases CPP and improves CBF. In addition, vasoconstriction in normal tissue and failure of autoregulation in damaged tissue divert blood flow to injured brain relieving ischaemia. Unfortunately, raised CCP eventually increases oedema and ICP in damaged brain and excess vasoconstriction may cause ischaemia in normal tissue. Consequently, a low-normal P_aCO_2 (~35–40mmHg) is currently recommended.

Immediate management

Requires: (i) **prompt resuscitation** with supplemental oxygen to correct hypoxia and ventilatory support to prevent hypercapnia. Intravenous fluids and antiarrhythmics maintain BP, CPP and haemodynamic stability; (ii) **spinal immobilization:** Assume all head-injured patients have cervical/spinal injuries; (iii) **airways protection** in obtunded patients. If intubation is necessary, stabilize the cervical spine with 'in-line' traction; (iv) **detection of other injuries:** ~50% have potentially lethal thoracic or abdominal injuries; and (v) **sedation (± paralysis)** to prevent ICP elevation and spinal injury in agitated patients.

Assessment

The **Glasgow Coma Score (GCS)**, a prognostic, reproducible method of assessing patient responsiveness (Fig. c). Severe head injury is defined as a GCS ≤ 8; postresuscitation GCS ≤ 8 within 48h of injury; or any intracranial contusion, haematoma or laceration.
• **Physical examination** detects head wounds and spinal cord damage. Basilar skull fractures are recognized as CSF rhinorrhoea, blood behind the tympanic membrane, 'racoon eyes' or

bruising behind the ears (Battle's sign). Papilloedema indicates raised ICP. Neurological examination is essential.
• **Radiographic evaluation** includes skull radiographs and/or CT scan (Fig. b). Immediate CT scan is indicated during coma or for deteriorating consciousness, GCS ≤ 8, GCS 9–13 with skull fractures, or planned surgery. Intracranial haematoma is 10-fold more common following skull fractures.
• **Monitoring.** GCS is adequate in mild injuries. Severe head injury may require **ICP monitoring** using extradural, subarachnoid space or direct brain tissue (e.g. Camino bolt) pressure transducers. Infection risks and inaccuracy limit use. **Cerebral oxygen saturation (S_jO_2)** is measured using a jugular venous bulb fibreoptic catheter. $S_jO_2 < 55\%$ suggests inadequate CBF. **Blood sugar** (BS) is monitored and occasionally **EEG**.

Management

Management aims to prevent secondary cerebral damage.
• **General measures** include optimizing CBF (i.e. MAP > 70mmHg, ICP < 15–20mmHg, CPP > 60mmHg) and oxygenation (i.e. $P_aO_2 > 90\%$ and $S_jO_2 > 55\%$).
• **Reduce ICP.** Therapeutic options are: (i) **hyperventilation** (P_aCO_2 25–30mmHg) which rapidly (~30s) reduces ICP (~25%) but prophylactic hyperventilation is not recommended as excessive vasoconstriction may impair CBF (see above); (ii) **loop diuretics (e.g. furosemide) and osmotic agents (e.g. mannitol)** which produce marked but transient ICP reductions (~6–8h) which may prevent cerebral herniation. Mannitol increases intravascular osmotic pressure and resulting fluid shifts reduce brain cell volume and ICP; (iii) **improved venous drainage:** Hard collars, neck flexion and tracheostomy ties can impede venous drainage and increase ICP. Midline head position with 15–30° elevation optimizes drainage. Suctioning, physiotherapy and PEEP increase venous pressure and should be minimized; (iv) **ventriculostomy drainage and decompressive surgery** which are indicated when other methods have failed. CSF drainage from the ventricles is particularly useful in obstructive hydrocephalus; and (v) **steroids** do not reduce ICP or improve outcome.
• **Reduce cerebral metabolism.** Therapeutic strategies include: (i) **tight glycaemic control** (BS 4–7 mmol/L) which improves outcome by reducing cerebral lactate production associated with hyperglycaemia; (ii) **prophylactic anticonvulsants** which prevent seizures that complicate ~10–40% of severe head injuries; (iii) **sedation and paralysis** which decrease agitation and metabolism. Propofol may be neuroprotective. **Barbiturates** (e.g. thiopentone) which reduce cerebral metabolic demand but cause haemodynamic instability. Benzodiazepines are a good alternative; and (iv) **preventing hyperthermia,** which damages injured brain, with antipyretics and cooling. Moderate hypothermia (33–34°C) may be neuroprotective.
• **Correct complications** associated with head injury (Fig. g). Avoid transnasal tubes in basilar skull fractures and treat signs of meningitis with antibiotics.

Prognosis

Road safety measures (e.g. seat belts, helmets, drink-driving legislation) have reduced head injury-related deaths. Nevertheless, in the USA, ~50000 severely head-injured patients (GCS ≤ 8) die before reaching hospital and ~50000 after hospital admission. Of survivors with an initial GCS ≤ 8, ~33% will never regain independent function, whereas ~66% will be largely independent.

46 Chest trauma

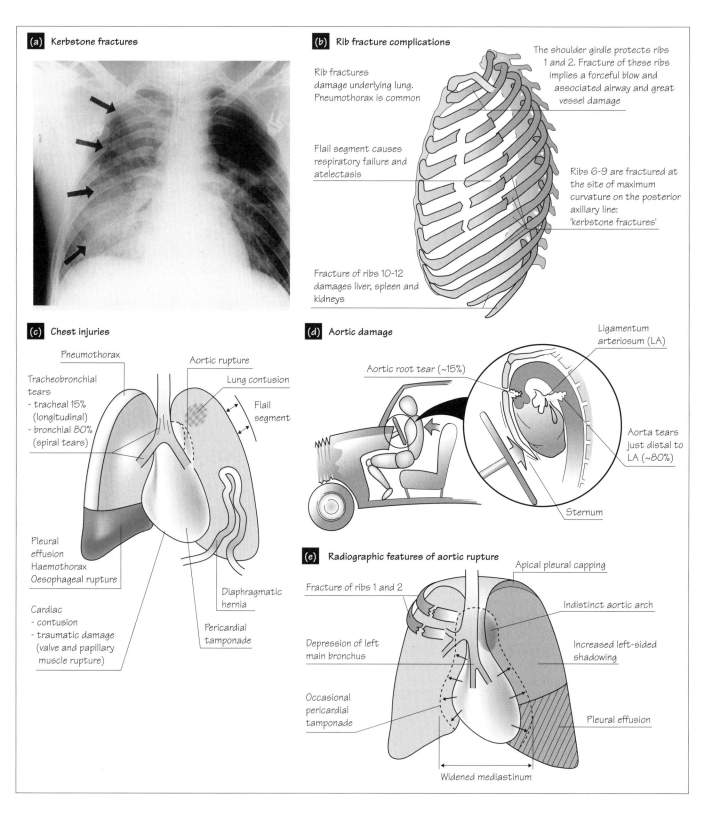

(a) Kerbstone fractures

(b) Rib fracture complications

Rib fractures damage underlying lung. Pneumothorax is common

Flail segment causes respiratory failure and atelectasis

Fracture of ribs 10-12 damages liver, spleen and kidneys

The shoulder girdle protects ribs 1 and 2. Fracture of these ribs implies a forceful blow and associated airway and great vessel damage

Ribs 6-9 are fractured at the site of maximum curvature on the posterior axillary line: 'kerbstone fractures'

(c) Chest injuries

Pneumothorax

Tracheobronchial tears
- tracheal 15% (longitudinal)
- bronchial 80% (spiral tears)

Pleural effusion
Haemothorax
Oesophageal rupture

Cardiac
- contusion
- traumatic damage (valve and papillary muscle rupture)

Aortic rupture

Lung contusion

Flail segment

Diaphragmatic hernia

Pericardial tamponade

(d) Aortic damage

Aortic root tear (~15%)

Ligamentum arteriosum (LA)

Aorta tears just distal to LA (~80%)

Sternum

(e) Radiographic features of aortic rupture

Fracture of ribs 1 and 2

Depression of left main bronchus

Occasional pericardial tamponade

Apical pleural capping

Indistinct aortic arch

Increased left-sided shadowing

Pleural effusion

Widened mediastinum

Chest trauma may be penetrating or blunt. It is often in associated with other injuries (Chapters 44, 45), some of which may require immediate surgery. Early correction of the hypoxaemia, hyper-capnia and hypotension that frequently accompany chest trauma prevents further damage (Chapters 4, 5, 44). Subsequent management involves monitoring for complications and missed injuries.

Penetrating chest trauma

• **Stab (e.g. knife) and low-velocity gunshot wounds** cause haemopneumothorax. Management with chest drainage alone will suffice in some patients. Indications for thoracotomy include a transmediastinal stab wound, cardiac tamponade, an initial blood loss of >1.5–2 L from the chest drains or persistent drainage of 200–250 mL/h which indicates ongoing bleeding from damaged blood vessels.

• **High-velocity gunshot wounds** cause extensive cavitation and tissue injury due to kinetic energy release. Early surgery is required to control haemorrhage or air leaks, evacuate blood clots and remove damaged lung. Air embolism may complicate any parenchymal lung damage but is more common in high-velocity gunshot wounds and during mechanical ventilation. It is suspected if neurological (e.g. CVA) or cardiac (e.g. arrhythmias) complications develop.

Blunt chest trauma

Non-penetrating blunt chest trauma is relatively common. There may be few external clinical signs apart from bruising. A high index of suspicion is required to avoid delayed diagnosis of serious internal injury. Three mechanisms cause intrathoracic injury.

1 *Rib fractures* (Figs a and b) damage underlying structures (e.g. pneumothorax, haemothorax, lung contusion) and cause severe pain with splinting, hypoventilation and atelectasis. They occur most frequently in older patients. In young patients chest wall flexibility results in intrathoracic damage without rib fractures. Treatment requires chest drainage, physiotherapy, potent analgesics including opioids, nerve blocks and epidural analgesia.

2 *Increased intrathoracic pressures.* Abrupt elevations of intracavitary pressure may rupture air- or fluid-filled structures. Oesophageal, alveolar and diaphragmatic rupture cause mediastinitis, pneumothorax and herniation of abdominal contents into the thoracic cavity, respectively (Fig. c).

3 *Shear stress.* Intrathoracic structures are tethered to adjacent tissues and shear forces produced by differential organ motion result in visceral or vascular tears including aortic rupture (Fig. d), tracheobronchial disruption and pulmonary haematoma.

Specific injuries

Tracheobronchial tears must be suspected when ribs 1 and 2 are fractured, with bilateral pneumothoraces or persistent air leaks. Characteristic sites of injury include longitudinal tears in the posterior membranous portion of the lower trachea (~15%) or spiral tears in the main bronchi (~80%). Bronchoscopy confirms the diagnosis and early surgical correction prevents atelectasis, infection and late development of bronchial stenosis and bronchiectasis. Occasionally a main bronchus is completely severed. The 'drop' lung is easily recognized and surgical repair is associated with no long-term complications.

Lung injuries (Fig. c) include:

• **Pneumothorax/haemothorax** which are frequent. Drainage is essential (Chapter 28).

• **Pulmonary contusions** with ill-defined infiltrates at the site of trauma on CXR. Haemoptysis and hypoxaemia are due to localized bleeding, oedema and associated V/Q mismatching.

• **Flail chest** which occurs when multiple fractures, usually at two sites, result in a free segment of chest wall or sternum. 'Paradoxi-cal' motion during normal breathing (i.e. segment moves in during inspiration and out during expiration) causes hypoventilation beneath the free segment with subsequent atelectasis. Discomfort also impedes chest wall movement and cough, further limiting ventilation and secretion clearance. Pain control is essential and thoracic epidural is the most effective technique. Mechanical ventilation (±tracheostomy) for ~7–14 days is required if respiratory failure develops (Chapter 10). This restores normal movement of the flail segment during inspiration/expiration. External chest wall stabilization (e.g. fixation, taping) is of no benefit.

• **Diaphragmatic injuries** which occur in ~7% of severe blunt chest injury, mostly on the left (~80%) as the right diaphragm is protected by the liver. Mortality is high because of associated splenic or hepatic rupture.

• **Lung torsion** which is rare.

Heart and great vessel injuries include:

• **Cardiac contusion** which causes local oedema and microvascular haemorrhage at the site of cardiac impact resulting in myocardial ischaemia, arrhythmias, heart block and ventricular failure. Cardiac enzymes, ECG, echocardiography and occasionally angiography or myocardial perfusion scans establish the diagnosis. Treatment is non-specific, including management of arrhythmias and circulatory failure (Chapters 5, 19, 20).

• **Aortic tears and dissection** which are due to shear stresses associated with abrupt deceleration accidents (e.g. car crashes; Fig. d). Most cases are fatal at the scene of the accident. Clinically there may be no evidence of external trauma and rib fractures are not always present. Tears are most common just distal to the *ligamentum arteriosum* (~80%). Tears of the aortic root (~15%) occasionally damage the aortic valve or coronary arteries. Figure (e) illustrates CXR features of aortic rupture. Angiography or contrast CT scans confirm the diagnosis.

• **Pericardial tamponade** which may be due to aortic root disruption, coronary artery laceration or rupture of the free ventricular wall. It usually requires surgical intervention.

• **Traumatic damage** which may involve the heart, valves (~60% aortic, ~30% mitral), papillary muscles or pericardium. Transmural rupture is rapidly fatal in >80% of cases. Early surgical repair is often required.

Oesophageal rupture is suspected if major trauma is associated with rapidly developing pleural effusion, pneumothorax or empyema. Aspirated pleural fluid often contains food particles and a raised amylase. Oesophageal barium studies confirm the diagnosis whereas endoscopy and CT scanning are often unhelpful. Prognosis is poor and mediastinitis is the most frequent cause of death.

Fat embolism syndrome occurs 1 h to 3 days after multiple longbone or pelvic fractures. Lipases hydrolyse triglycerides, liberating fatty acids into the circulation which are toxic to the lung. In addition, small fat emboli pass through the pulmonary capillaries to affect retinal, skin and CNS vessels. The characteristic clinical triad includes **confusion, pulmonary dysfunction** (e.g. cough, dyspnoea, pleurisy and ARDS) and a **petechial skin rash** over the upper torso. Coagulopathy (e.g. DIC) may also occur. Investigations reveal hypoxaemia, a normal early CXR and lipase and fat globules in urine and serum.

47 Acute abdominal emergencies

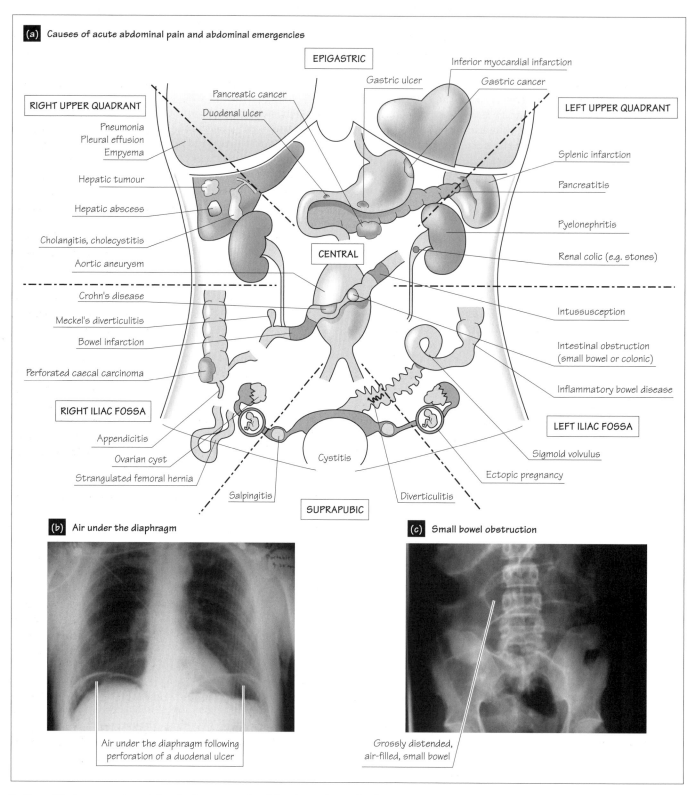

(a) Causes of acute abdominal pain and abdominal emergencies

EPIGASTRIC

Inferior myocardial infarction

Gastric ulcer

Gastric cancer

RIGHT UPPER QUADRANT

Pancreatic cancer

Duodenal ulcer

LEFT UPPER QUADRANT

Pneumonia
Pleural effusion
Empyema

Splenic infarction

Pancreatitis

Hepatic tumour

Hepatic abscess

Pyelonephritis

Cholangitis, cholecystitis

Renal colic (e.g. stones)

Aortic aneurysm

CENTRAL

Crohn's disease

Intussusception

Meckel's diverticulitis

Bowel infarction

Intestinal obstruction
(small bowel or colonic)

Perforated caecal carcinoma

Inflammatory bowel disease

RIGHT ILIAC FOSSA

Appendicitis

LEFT ILIAC FOSSA

Ovarian cyst

Cystitis

Sigmoid volvulus

Strangulated femoral hernia

Ectopic pregnancy

Salpingitis

Diverticulitis

SUPRAPUBIC

(b) Air under the diaphragm

Air under the diaphragm following
perforation of a duodenal ulcer

(c) Small bowel obstruction

Grossly distended,
air-filled, small bowel

In the critical care setting, abdominal emergencies (Fig. a) rarely present with typical symptoms and signs. Coma, spinal cord injury or drugs (e.g. sedatives, analgesics) mask many characteristic features (e.g. rebound tenderness in peritonitis). Relatively minor findings including feeding intolerance, diarrhoea and vague abdominal discomfort may be the only indicators of abdominal pathology. Early diagnosis requires a low threshold of suspicion, repeated abdominal examination, monitoring of vital signs (e.g.

temperature, BP) and timely investigation (e.g. amylase, WCC, radiography). CT scans provide optimal imaging but USSs are portable and readily detect liver, renal and pelvic abnormalities. Avoid excessive use of analgesia before diagnosis, involve surgeons early in evaluation and withhold feeding if laparotomy may be required. Non-abdominal pathology (e.g. inferior MI) presenting with abdominal features must be excluded. Many abdominal emergencies are complicated by peritonitis, bacteraemia and subsequent multiple organ failure (Chapter 16).

- **Peptic ulcer perforation** complicates duodenal (5–10%) rather than gastric (<1%) ulcers. It occurs at any age but is most common between 20 and 40 years. There may be no previous history of peptic ulcer disease. Perforation usually presents as sudden, severe mid-abdominal pain. Patients appear ill, lie still and take shallow breaths to minimize pain. Examination reveals a rigid, 'board-like' abdomen and absent bowel sounds. Older patients on steroids or NSAIDs and critically ill patients may not exhibit peritonitis. An erect CXR (Fig. b) or left lateral decubitus view of the abdomen detects free air in the abdominal cavity (~80%).

Management includes fluid resuscitation, antibiotics and nasogastric (NG) tube drainage. In unstable patients, duodenal ulcers are oversewn, whereas resection and vagotomy may be indicated in stable patients. Whenever possible, gastric ulcers are resected because of associated carcinoma risk (Chapter 34).

- **Small bowel obstruction** (SBO) may be simple or associated with vascular compromise (e.g. volvulus). It presents with nausea, vomiting, cramping abdominal pain and distension. Initially bowel sounds are high pitched ('tinkling') but become infrequent with prolonged obstruction. Adhesions from previous surgery cause ~75% of SBO and incarcerated hernias, malignancy and volvulus ~25%. Intussusception, gallstones and inflammatory bowel disease (IBD) are less common. Upright or decubitus abdominal radiographs demonstrate dilated small bowel (>3 cm) with or without air–fluid levels (Fig. c).

Conservative management involves fluid and electrolyte resuscitation and gastric decompression with NG tube suction.

Surgery is indicated if symptoms persist or the clinical condition fails to improve after 24 h (i.e. fever, tachycardia). Following abdominal surgery prolonged ileus may mimic SBO and a longer trial of decompression is necessary.

- **Colonic obstruction** (±perforation) usually affects the elderly. It presents with acute abdominal pain, vomiting (~50%), constipation (~50%) and distension. Colonic cancer, diverticular disease, sigmoid volvulus and faecal impaction are common causes. Pseudo-obstruction with colonic dilation (±caecal perforation) can develop in the absence of a mechanical cause due to electrolyte imbalance, myxoedema, anticholinergic drugs or medical debility. Toxic megacolon (±perforation) occurs in severe ulcerative colitis. Plain radiographs are often diagnostic, demonstrating colonic distension, volvulus or subdiaphragmatic air following perforation. An acute increase in caecal diameter to >9 cm suggests imminent perforation.

Conservative management includes colonic decompression by rectal tube or colonoscopy, electrolyte correction and discontinuation of sedative or narcotic agents.

Surgery. Imminent caecal perforation requires decompressive caecostomy. A limited right hemicolectomy, ileostomy and mucous fistula are recommended following perforation.

- **Mesenteric ischaemia** affects elderly patients with heart and vascular disease. Mortality is ~70%. Superior mesenteric artery (SMA) occlusion causes ~50% of acute bowel ischaemia (ABI). It presents with severe abdominal pain and leucocytosis but few physical signs. Inferior mesenteric artery (IMA) occlusion has a more subtle presentation and causes ~25% of ABI. Acute proximal SMA and IMA thrombosis is usually due to atherosclerosis. Slow occlusion can be accompanied by intestinal angina (i.e. pain after meals). Embolic occlusion occurs with atrial fibrillation or post-MI mural thrombosis. Less common causes of occlusive ischaemia include vasculitis and mesenteric venous thrombosis. Non-occlusive infarction due to hypotension, cardiac failure or vasopressor drugs is increasingly recognized in critically ill patients. Initially ABI produces oedematous mucosal injury with occult blood or bloody diarrhoea in ~50% of cases. Mucosal sloughing, bowel necrosis, perforation, peritonitis, sepsis, shock and death follow. Refractory metabolic (lactic) acidosis with hyperkalaemia is characteristic.

Management includes resuscitation, antibiotics and electrolyte correction. In selected cases angiography confirms the diagnosis, allows vasodilator infusion (e.g. nitroglycerin) and may aid surgical revascularization.

Surgery to resect gangrenous bowel is essential in patients with peritoneal signs. Re-exploration at 24–36 h allows demarcation and further resection of non-viable tissue. Unfortunately, delayed diagnosis or extensive infarction usually renders the clinical situation hopeless.

- **Cholecystitis and cholangitis** are normally due to gallstone obstruction of the cystic duct (~90%). In critically ill patients, acalculous cholecystitis is common due to biliary reflux or cholestasis following loss of feeding-induced gallbladder emptying. In these patients, biliary-associated sepsis is often overlooked. The classical triad of fever, rigors and right upper quadrant (RUQ) pain occurs in ~70%. Additional features include leucocytosis (~70%), vomiting, RUQ mass (~20%) and elevated bilirubin, alkaline phosphatase and amylase (in the absence of pancreatitis). Ultrasonography and CT scans may demonstrate a dilated biliary tract due to gallstones. A dilated gallbladder (>5 cm), thickened wall (>3 mm), sediment and pericholecystic fluid collections are suggestive of acalculous cholecystitis. Common infective organisms are *E. coli*, *Klebsiella*, *Streptococcus faecalis* and anaerobes.

Management includes resuscitation, analgesics, broad-spectrum antibiotics and biliary drainage. In critically ill patients, the simplest procedure is indicated, with reoperation when stability is achieved. T-tube drainage of the biliary tract (±cholecystectomy) is effective. Percutaneous drainage is an option in high-risk patients but may cause potentially lethal bile peritonitis.

- **Other acute abdominal emergencies** must be excluded, including pancreatitis (Chapter 36), ruptured or leaking aortic aneurysms, pelvic disease in females (e.g. pelvic inflammatory disease, ectopic pregnancy, ovarian torsion), appendicitis, retroperitoneal haematoma (e.g. renal trauma) and renal calculi.

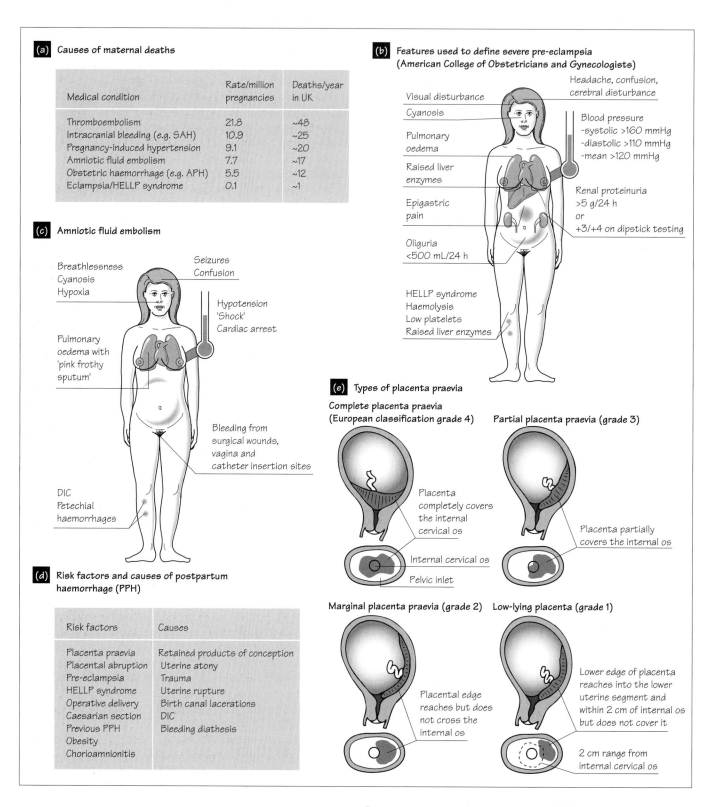

(a) Causes of maternal deaths

Medical condition	Rate/million pregnancies	Deaths/year in UK
Thromboembolism	21.8	~48
Intracranial bleeding (e.g. SAH)	10.9	~25
Pregnancy-induced hypertension	9.1	~20
Amniotic fluid embolism	7.7	~17
Obstetric haemorrhage (e.g. APH)	5.5	~12
Eclampsia/HELLP syndrome	0.1	~1

(b) Features used to define severe pre-eclampsia (American College of Obstetricians and Gynecologists)

Headache, confusion, cerebral disturbance
Visual disturbance
Cyanosis
Pulmonary oedema
Raised liver enzymes
Epigastric pain
Oliguria <500 mL/24 h
Blood pressure
-systolic >160 mmHg
-diastolic >110 mmHg
-mean >120 mmHg
Renal proteinuria >5 g/24 h or +3/+4 on dipstick testing
HELLP syndrome
Haemolysis
Low platelets
Raised liver enzymes

(c) Amniotic fluid embolism

Breathlessness
Cyanosis
Hypoxia
Seizures
Confusion
Hypotension 'Shock' Cardiac arrest
Pulmonary oedema with 'pink frothy sputum'
Bleeding from surgical wounds, vagina and catheter insertion sites
DIC Petechial haemorrhages

(d) Risk factors and causes of postpartum haemorrhage (PPH)

Risk factors	Causes
Placenta praevia	Retained products of conception
Placental abruption	Uterine atony
Pre-eclampsia	Trauma
HELLP syndrome	Uterine rupture
Operative delivery	Birth canal lacerations
Caesarian section	DIC
Previous PPH	Bleeding diathesis
Obesity	
Chorioamnionitis	

(e) Types of placenta praevia

Complete placenta praevia (European classification grade 4)
Placenta completely covers the internal cervical os
Internal cervical os
Pelvic inlet

Partial placenta praevia (grade 3)
Placenta partially covers the internal os

Marginal placenta praevia (grade 2)
Placental edge reaches but does not cross the internal os

Low-lying placenta (grade 1)
Lower edge of placenta reaches into the lower uterine segment and within 2 cm of internal os but does not cover it
2 cm range from internal cervical os

Life-threatening obstetric emergencies occur antepartum and postpartum. In the developed world, maternal and fetal mortality has decreased dramatically but avoidable deaths continue to occur. Table (a) reports the main causes and associated death rates.

Pregnancy-induced hypertension (PIH) or pre-eclampsia

PIH or pre-eclampsia is defined as 'gestational hypertension with proteinuria developing during pregnancy or labour'. Placental delivery is the only cure. PIH affects ~10% of pregnancies, usually between 32 and 38 weeks' gestation and resolves 2–3 days after delivery. Any of the features in Fig. (b) are used to define severe PIH. Eclampsia is diagnosed if grand mal convulsions occur. Cerebral oedema, ARDS, pulmonary oedema, intracranial haemorrhage or liver damage may cause death.

Management aims to prevent vasospasm, improve perfusion of the uterus, placenta and vital organs and assess fetal maturity.

• **Antihypertensive therapy** (e.g. nifedipine, labetalol) is required if diastolic pressure is persistently > 100 mmHg.

• **Fluid therapy.** Assessing fluid requirements is difficult as CVP correlates poorly with left heart pressures. Left atrial pressure measurement (Chapter 2) is indicated during transfusions, prolonged oliguria or pulmonary oedema.

• **Monitor** urine output, proteinuria, liver function, platelet count and urate.

• **Magnesium sulphate** may be given as prophylaxis against convulsions. It is a CNS depressant, cerebral vasodilator and mild antihypertensive. Therapeutic blood levels are 2–3 mmol/L but respiratory rate, S_aO_2, ECG and mental status are monitored because respiratory paralysis and heart block occur at 7–8 mmol/L. In overdose, magnesium can be inhibited by calcium gluconate.

• **Fetal assessment.** Early fetal delivery may be required. If the pregnancy is <34 weeks, dexamethasone aids fetal lung maturation. Delivery is delayed for 48 h for maximum benefit.

Amniotic fluid embolism (AFE)

AFE affects 1 in 10–80 000 pregnancies. It occurs when amniotic fluid or fetal matter (e.g. meconium) enters the maternal circulation. It frequently affects older, multiparous mothers with large babies during oxytocin-driven labour. Less commonly it occurs during amniocentesis, termination, abdominal trauma, caesarian section (CS) or artificial membrane rupture. Figure (c) illustrates the clinical features. Sudden breathlessness, cyanosis and hypotension may be followed by cardiac arrest. Initial survivors develop seizures (~20%), DIC with bleeding (~40%) and non-cardiogenic pulmonary oedema (~75%). Management is symptomatic (e.g. oxygen) and supportive (e.g. ventilation). Mortality can be >80% with ~50% dying within the first hour.

Major haemorrhage

Blood loss >40% during pregnancy is life-threatening. Resuscitation follows the guidelines used for any major blood loss (Chapters 4, 41). Obstetric intervention depends on the cause.

1 *Antepartum haemorrhage (APH)* is bleeding from the birth canal after the 20th week of pregnancy that puts the fetus at risk. The main causes are placental abruption (~25%), placenta praevia (~20%), uterine rupture and placental abnormalities (e.g. vasa praevia). Ultrasound scans determine the cause.

• **Placental abruption** is due to haemorrhage into the decidua basalis with placental separation. Hypertensive disorders, trauma and sudden changes in uterine size are potential precipitating factors but usually there is no obvious cause. It affects ~1.5% of pregnancies and is more common in smokers, low socioecomomic groups and older, multiparous women. Bleeding may be concealed, revealed or both. With increasing placental separation there is abdominal pain and tenderness. The uterine fundus may be higher than expected for gestational age. Retroplacental bleeding >500 mL may cause fetal death due to reduced func-

tional intervillous space, vasoconstriction and uterine spasm; >1 L bleeding causes maternal shock and DIC.

• **Placenta praevia (PP)** affects ~1% of pregnancies. It occurs when the placenta lies in the lower uterine segment (LUS). The greater the placental encroachment on the os, the higher the maternal morbidity and mortality (Fig. e). The LUS endometrium is less well developed and placental attachment to underlying muscle (PP accreta) impairs separation during delivery. Painless vaginal bleeding in late pregnancy is regarded as PP until proved otherwise. Patients with PP and APH are hospitalized in later pregnancy but management is conservative to allow fetal maturation. Delivery by CS is usually required. Haemorrhage may occur and blood must be cross-matched prior to surgery.

2 *Primary postpartum haemorrhage (PPH)* describes bleeding of >500 mL from the birth canal in the first 24 h after delivery and is considered severe if >1 L/24 h. Risk factors and causes are listed in Table (d).

• **Retained products of conception (RPC)** affect ~4% of pregnancies and require uterine evacuation. Severe haemorrhage may entail embolization, iliac artery ligation or hysterectomy.

• **Uterine rupture** occurs in multiparous women with fetal malpresentations, operative trauma, breech delivery, PP accreta or oxytocin use.

• **Uterine atony** is due to drugs (e.g. β-blockers), uterine sepsis, bladder distension, multiparity or long labour and is uncommon since the advent of oxytocic drugs. Treatments include uterine massage, bimanual compression, oxytocin, uterine packing or intramyometrial prostaglandin.

• **Coagulation defects** occur following abruption, intrauterine death, pre-eclampsia, sepsis or AFE.

3 *Secondary PPH* is excessive bleeding >24 h postpartum until the end of the puerperium. It is usually due to infected RPC and is treated with antibiotics.

Sheehan's syndrome is panhypopituitarism following pituitary hypoperfusion during severe obstetric haemorrhage. Early manifestations are lactation failure and amenorrhoea. Adrenal and thyroid gland failure follow (Chapter 33).

Medical emergencies in pregnancy

Cardiac arrest in pregnancy. Advanced life support guidelines are followed (Chapter 21). Early intubation is essential because reduced pulmonary compliance (i.e. diaphragmatic splinting) and increased oxygen consumption cause rapid hypoxaemia. Chest compressions are performed with a wedge below the right hip or manual uterine displacement to prevent caval compression which impairs venous return. Immediate fetal delivery is required if resuscitation is unsuccessful. Resuscitation continues until after delivery by CS. Gastric compression makes aspiration a risk.

Pulmonary thromboembolism (PE) (Chapter 27) is the **commonest cause** of maternal deaths and affects ~1 in 2000 pregnancies. Caval compression by the gravid uterus and pregnancy-induced clotting factor changes predispose to antepartum lower limb and pelvic venous thrombosis. Mobilization after delivery may precipitate PE.

Intracranial bleeds are primary or due to subarachnoid haemorrhage.

49 Burns, toxic inhalation and electrical injuries

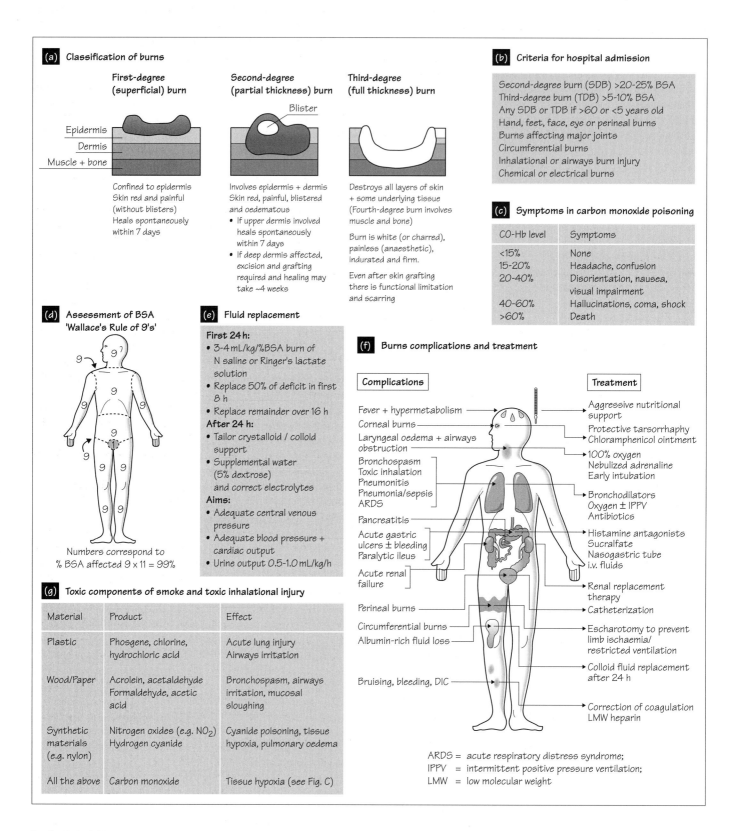

(a) Classification of burns

First-degree (superficial) burn

Epidermis
Dermis
Muscle + bone

Confined to epidermis
Skin red and painful
(without blisters)
Heals spontaneously
within 7 days

Second-degree (partial thickness) burn

Blister

Involves epidermis + dermis
Skin red, painful, blistered
and oedematous
- If upper dermis involved
  heals spontaneously
  within 7 days
- If deep dermis affected,
  excision and grafting
  required and healing may
  take ~4 weeks

Third-degree (full thickness) burn

Destroys all layers of skin
+ some underlying tissue
(Fourth-degree burn involves
muscle and bone)

Burn is white (or charred),
painless (anaesthetic),
indurated and firm.

Even after skin grafting
there is functional limitation
and scarring

(b) Criteria for hospital admission

Second-degree burn (SDB) >20-25% BSA
Third-degree burn (TDB) >5-10% BSA
Any SDB or TDB if >60 or <5 years old
Hand, feet, face, eye or perineal burns
Burns affecting major joints
Circumferential burns
Inhalational or airways burn injury
Chemical or electrical burns

(c) Symptoms in carbon monoxide poisoning

CO-Hb level	Symptoms
<15%	None
15-20%	Headache, confusion
20-40%	Disorientation, nausea, visual impairment
40-60%	Hallucinations, coma, shock
>60%	Death

(d) Assessment of BSA 'Wallace's Rule of 9's'

9
9
9
9
9
9
9
9
9
9
9
1

Numbers correspond to
% BSA affected 9 x 11 = 99%

(e) Fluid replacement

First 24 h:
- 3-4 mL/kg/%BSA burn of
  N saline or Ringer's lactate
  solution
- Replace 50% of deficit in first
  8 h
- Replace remainder over 16 h

After 24 h:
- Tailor crystalloid / colloid
  support
- Supplemental water
  (5% dextrose)
  and correct electrolytes

Aims:
- Adequate central venous
  pressure
- Adequate blood pressure +
  cardiac output
- Urine output 0.5-1.0 mL/kg/h

(f) Burns complications and treatment

Complications

Fever + hypermetabolism
Corneal burns
Laryngeal oedema + airways
obstruction
Bronchospasm
Toxic inhalation
Pneumonitis
Pneumonia/sepsis
ARDS
Pancreatitis
Acute gastric
ulcers ± bleeding
Paralytic ileus
Acute renal
failure
Perineal burns
Circumferential burns
Albumin-rich fluid loss

Bruising, bleeding, DIC

Treatment

Aggressive nutritional
support
Protective tarsorrhaphy
Chloramphenicol ointment
100% oxygen
Nebulized adrenaline
Early intubation
Bronchodilators
Oxygen ± IPPV
Antibiotics
Histamine antagonists
Sucralfate
Nasogastric tube
i.v. fluids
Renal replacement
therapy
Catheterization
Escharotomy to prevent
limb ischaemia/
restricted ventilation
Colloid fluid replacement
after 24 h
Correction of coagulation
LMW heparin

ARDS = acute respiratory distress syndrome;
IPPV = intermittent positive pressure ventilation;
LMW = low molecular weight

(g) Toxic components of smoke and toxic inhalational injury

Material	Product	Effect
Plastic	Phosgene, chlorine, hydrochloric acid	Acute lung injury Airways irritation
Wood/Paper	Acrolein, acetaldehyde Formaldehyde, acetic acid	Bronchospasm, airways irritation, mucosal sloughing
Synthetic materials (e.g. nylon)	Nitrogen oxides (e.g. NO_2) Hydrogen cyanide	Cyanide poisoning, tissue hypoxia, pulmonary oedema
All the above	Carbon monoxide	Tissue hypoxia (see Fig. C)

In the UK, 200 000 people suffer with burns each year, 10 000 are admitted to hospital and ~500 die. Mortality is decreasing and patients may survive burns >90% body surface area (BSA). Old age and lower socioeconomic group are predictors of increased mortality.

Assessment of burns

- **Depth** is classified according to the skin layers affected, appearance and healing (Fig. a) as **first-degree** (superficial), **second-degree** (partial-thickness) or **third-degree** (full-thickness) burns.
- **BSA affected** is estimated by the 'rule of nines' in adults (Fig. d).
- **Cause** may be dry (e.g. flame), moist (e.g. hot liquids), blast, electrical or chemical.
- **Time** allows assessment of when fluid resuscitation should have started.
- **Site affected.** Face (e.g. eyelids), perineum, hands, feet and circumferential burns require specialist attention.
- **Smoke inhalation.** Frequent in enclosed spaces and associated with increased mortality.

Management of major burns

Figure (b) defines major burns requiring hospital admission and/or referral to specialist centres. Figure (f) illustrates complications of burns injury.

1 *Resuscitation.* Burns activate the inflammatory cascade causing increased vascular permeability. Hypovolaemia and shock develop rapidly due to fluid shifts (i.e intravascular to extravascular) and exudation through injured skin. Immediate fluid replacement is required for burns >20% BSA (>15% with smoke inhalation) to maintain organ function and preserve viable skin tissue by restoring perfusion.

- **First 24h:** crystalloid-only regimes are usually used. Colloid and hypertonic solutions do not improve outcome. The Parkland formula recommends 3–4 mL/kg/%BSA burn/day of normal saline or Ringer's solution, with 50% given in the first 8h (Fig. e). Fluid requirements must also be titrated against clinical, haemodynamic and urinary output parameters. All fluid replacement strategies cause tissue oedema; however, hypertonic saline may produce less oedema in non-burnt tissue.
- **After 24h:** sodium requirements and vessel permeability decrease. Low sodium solutions and colloids are used to maintain circulating volume and electrolyte balance.

Vasoactive agents may be required (e.g. sepsis) but avoid α-adrenergic agonists (e.g. norepinephrine) as these decrease blood flow to injured skin.

2 *Airway complications* often cause early death. Presence of facial/neck burns, oropharyngeal swelling, cough, carbonaceous sputum, respiratory distress or stridor suggests upper airway damage and inhalational injury. Hyperventilation and hypercapnia due to increased metabolism may also cause respiratory failure.

- **Airways obstruction.** Hot gases (e.g. steam) and toxic compounds in smoke cause rapid upper airways obstruction. Early intubation is recommended in second- or third-degree facial burns, as this may be impossible later due to oedema. If intubation is not required, monitor for obstruction (i.e. pulmonary function tests) and give humidified oxygen and nebulized bronchodilators (±ephedrine). Steroids do not reduce oedema and increase infection risks.
- **Toxic inhalational injury (TII).** Highly soluble gases (e.g. SO_2, Cl) dissolve in upper airway secretions forming potent acids which cause mucosal inflammation, ulceration and bronchospasm (Table g). Low-solubility toxins (e.g. NO_2, phosgene) penetrate to the lower respiratory tract, causing alveolar damage, pulmonary oedema and V/Q mismatch. In severe TII, mucosa sloughs at ~72h and requires 7–14 days to regenerate. Infection and pneumonitis are common during this time.
- **Carbon monoxide (CO) poisoning** causes 75% of fire fatalities. Affinity of CO for Hb is ~250 times that of oxygen. Low CO levels (i.e. 0.1%) rapidly displace oxygen to produce non-functional carboxyhaemoglobin (CO-Hb). Symptoms of CO poisoning are those of tissue hypoxia (Table c) and correlate with CO-Hb levels. Co-oximeters with multiwavelength spectroscopy differentiate between CO-Hb and oxyhaemoglobin. Pulse oximeters cannot do this and record inappropriately high saturations. Treatment with 100% oxygen decreases the half-life of CO-Hb from 180 to 30min and is continued until the CO-Hb is <10%. Hyperbaric oxygen therapy may reduce neuropsychiatric sequelae in patients with CO-Hb levels >30%. Transport difficulties usually outweigh benefits.
- **Cyanide (CN) poisoning** causes histotoxic hypoxia. In smoke inhalation, lactic acid levels correlate with CN levels. Persisting metabolic acidosis requires treatment with sodium thiosulphite which speeds hepatic metabolism or dicobalt edetate which binds CN to form an inactive complex.

3 *Metabolism and nutrition.* Increased basal metabolic rate, reflected by fever (~38.5°C) and hypercapnia, peaks at ~7 days and is proportional to burn size and associated infection. High environmental temperatures (e.g. ~32°C ± high humidity) reduce heat and water loss and calorie expenditure. Early enteral feeding is recommended. The large calorie requirements are calculated from burn size. Prophylactic H_2 antagonists (e.g. ranitidine) reduce the high incidence of stress ulceration.

4 *Burn wound care and skin grafts.* Early debridement and skin grafting improve functional outcome and decrease infection, pain, healing time and mortality. Scalds are treated conservatively as they may heal without scarring. In massive burns (>60% BSA), inadequate donor sites may require the use of transplant or biosynthetic skins. Topical antibiotics (e.g. silver sulphadiazine, sodium nitrate) reduce early bacterial colonization with *Staphylococcus* and later Gram-negative rods (e.g. *Pseudomonas*).

5 *Infection.* Systemic antibiotics are reserved for documented wound infections (e.g. biopsy). Skin barrier loss and reduced immunity render patients susceptible to systemic infections. Pulmonary sepsis often causes death following severe burns, especially after smoke inhalation.

6 *Analgesia.* Initially intravenous opioids (e.g. morphine) are required. Ketamine provides long-lasting analgesia and is good for repeated dressing changes when combined with a benzodiazepine. Drug levels are monitored due to altered renal and hepatic clearance.

7 *Complications* (Fig. f). Circumferential contraction of neck, chest or limbs burns can cause life-threatening ventilatory impairment or distal limb ischaemia requiring immediate escharotomies.

Chemical and electrical burns

- **Chemical burns** are copiously irrigated with water and then treated like thermal burns. In acid or alkali burns avoid neutralizing solutions as exothermic reactions may cause additional thermal damage.
- **Electrical burns** (e.g. lightning, high voltage) produce extensive internal tissue damage and rhabdomyolysis with little external evidence of injury. Exit wounds (e.g. hands, feet) are often overlooked. Monitor for arrhythmias and myocardial injury.

Burns, toxic inhalation and electrical injuries

Appendix: Antiarrhythmic drugs

Classification of antiarrhythmic drugs (based on Vaughan Williams classification)

Class/examples	Mechanisms of action	Use
Class I:	All block Na$^+$ channels slowing depolarization + raising threshold for triggering impulses (AP). Drug dissociation rates from Na$^+$ channels vary; Class Ia ~5 s, Ib~500 ms, Ic~10–20 s	Slows conduction, suppresses re-entry + automaticity
Ia Disopyramide, quinidine	↑AP duration. ↑QT interval = ↑automaticity. ↑AVN conduction = ↑HR in AF	SVT + VT but must block AVN (e.g. digoxin) in AF
Ib Lignocaine, mexiletine	↓AP duration + greatly ↓conduction	VT especially after MI
Ic Flecainide	Greatly ↓conduction, no effect on AP duration but ↓contractility may cause hypotension	VT + some SVT (e.g. WPW syndrome)
Class II Atenolol, metoprolol	β-blockers act mainly on SAN: ↓spontaneous depolarization = ↓HR + ↓sympathetic drive (e.g. MI, stress) = ↓automaticity (↓ latent pacemakers)	SVT + VT especially after MI
Class III Amiodarone, sotalol,	Block K$^+$ channels. ↑AP duration by ↓repolarization. ↑QT interval risks automaticity (e.g. torsades de pointes). Also has class Ia, II + VI actions	SVT + VT. Most effective in re-entry tachycardias
Class IV Verapamil, diltiazem	Block Ca^{2+} slow channels, ↓nodal conduction + automaticity. Also ↓contractility + risks hypotension	SVT especially AVN re-entrant tachycardias
Other Classes Adenosine, digoxin	Adenosine acts on A$_1$-receptors + ↓Ca^{2+} / ↑K$^+$ currents to ↓AVN conduction. Digoxin ↓AVN conduction by vagal stimulation	Adenosine rapidly terminates + digoxin slows (± cardiovert) SVT

AP = action potential, AVN = atrioventricular node, AF = atrial fibrillation, WPW = Wolff-Parkinson-White, SAN = sinoatrial node, HR = heart rate, MI = myocardial infarction

Index

Note: page numbers in *italics* refer to figures.